The Southern Conference
on Gerontology

[Proceedings]

VOLUME 19
INSTITUTE OF GERONTOLOGY SERIES

(Communications relating to gerontology at the University of Florida should be addressed to Institute of Gerontology, 221 Matherly Hall, University of Florida, Gainesville, Florida 32601. This publication, and all previous publications of the University of Florida Institute of Gerontology, may be obtained from the University of Florida Press, Gainesville, Florida.)

Institute of Gerontology Series

Health Care Services

for the Aged

Problems in Effective Delivery and Use

Edited by
Carter C. Osterbind

Published for the
University of Florida Institute of Gerontology
by the
University of Florida Press
Gainesville, 1970

A University of Florida Press Book

Library of Congress Catalog Number 53-12339
ISBN 0–8130–0310–5

PRINTED BY STORTER PRINTING COMPANY, INCORPORATED
GAINESVILLE, FLORIDA

Registrants

Mrs. Harriet Agster
501 W. Davis Boulevard
Tampa, Florida 33606

Ruth E. Albrecht
Professor of Sociology
University of Florida
Gainesville, Florida 32601

Park Allen
615 S. Peninsula Drive
Daytona Beach, Florida 32018

Eleanor E. Armstrong
Pinellas County Nursing Home
250 Ulmerton Road
Largo, Florida 33540

George D. Barton
Administrator, Winter Park Towers
1111 South Lakemont Avenue
Winter Park, Florida 32789

M. A. Barton, M.D.
Mound Park Hospital Foundation,
  Inc.
St. Petersburg, Florida 33701

Mrs. M. A. Barton
Mound Park Hospital Foundation,
  Inc.
St. Petersburg, Florida 33701

Dexter Bates
Bishop Gray Inn
Box 668
Davenport, Florida 33837

Mrs. Dexter Bates
Bishop Gray Inn
Box 668
Davenport, Florida 33837

R. O. Beckman
Apt. 4
805 SW. 6th Street
Miami, Florida 33130

Gladys M. Biber
3939 SW. 5th Place
Gainesville, Florida 32601

Robert Bigelow
789 Don Mills Road
Toronto, Canada

Colon Blue
1661 Idle Drive
Clearwater, Florida 33510

Mrs. Thelma Bonner
112 Dolores Drive
Altermonte Springs, Florida 32701

Mrs. Mary K. Boyd
315 NE. 9th Street
Gainesville, Florida 32601

Mary V. Brown
Albany Junior College
2400 Gillionville Road
Albany, Georgia 31705

Harry R. Bryan
2414 Bull Street
Columbia, South Carolina 29201

v

Health Care Services for the Aged

Patty Ree Buchanan
Tennessee Commission on Aging
Capitol Towers
Nashville, Tennessee 37219

Fredric Buchholtz
Neighborly Center, Inc.
2350 22 Avenue South
St. Petersburg, Florida 33712

Adelaide K. Bullen
Florida State Museum
Seagle Building
University of Florida
Gainesville, Florida 32601

Mrs. Mable Butler
1820 Mirror Street
Orlando, Florida 32805

Mrs. Laura Caldwell
10 Nelson Avenue
DeFuniak Springs, Florida 32433

Pauline Calloway
Associate Professor
Extension Home Economist
University of Florida
Gainesville, Florida 32601

John M. Champion
Professor of Health and Hospital Administration
907 Lake Shore Towers
University of Florida
Gainesville, Florida 32601

Mary J. Clarke
1031 South Beach
Daytona Beach, Florida 32017

S. George Clark
P.O. Box 1147
Avon Park, Florida 33825

Pauline Council
Institute for Social Research
Florida State University
Tallahassee, Florida 32306

Francis W. Cox
1221 Nottingham
Orlando, Florida 32803

Lamar E. Crevasse, Jr.
Assistant Dean and Professor of Medicine
Box 746, Medical Science Building
University of Florida
Gainesville, Florida 32601

Janet Cuthrell
Winter Park Towers
1111 South Lakemont Avenue
Winter Park, Florida 32789

Franklin S. Cuyler
P.O. Box 1491
Lake Worth, Florida 33460

Mrs. Franklin S. Cuyler
P.O. Box 1491
Lake Worth, Florida 33460

Miss Beth Daane
Florida Library Association
1402 NW. 7th Avenue
Gainesville, Florida 32601

Charles M. Daly
Division of Family Services
P.O. Box 2050
Jacksonville, Florida 32201

R. A. Dauber
1216 E. Colonial
Orlando, Florida 32803

L. V. Davis
Department of Commerce
Caldwell Building
Tallahassee, Florida 32304

Marie K. Davis
2510 Central Avenue
St. Petersburg, Florida 33712

Samuel Demps
Housing Authority of Jacksonville
3550 Brentwood Ave.
Jacksonville, Florida 32206

Joseph DiBona
University of South Florida
Tampa, Florida 33620

Mrs. Emily Dickinson
915 South Rome
Tampa, Florida 33606

Dudley H. Dickson
University of South Florida
4114 Palmira Street
Tampa, Florida 33609

Michael J. Dougher
Salhaven Foundation, Inc.
P.O. Drawer 937
Jupiter, Florida 33458

E. Douglas Endsley
Community Service Council
1300 S. Andrews Avenue
Fort Lauderdale, Florida 33316

Sidney Entman
River Garden Hebrew Home for the
Aged
1800 Stockton Street
Jacksonville, Florida 32204

J. M. Farris
1531 Wellington Road
Birmingham, Alabama 35209

Selma C. Fimbel
157 Central Avenue
St. Petersburg, Florida 33711

Viola Fischer, M.D.
Memorial Home Community
Penney Farms, Florida 32079

Miss Louise Flowers
315 Riverside Avenue
Jacksonville, Florida 32202

Virginia C. Fountain
6562 Lou Drive, North
Jacksonville, Florida 32216

Floyd J. Fowler
Joint Center for Urban Studies
Cambridge, Massachusetts 02138

Mrs. Dorothy Fox
1031 South Beach
Daytona Beach, Florida 32017

Signe E. Froberg
Florida Regional Medical Program
1 Davis Boulevard
Tampa, Florida 33606

Jesse J. Fuller
307 Ashley Drive
Tampa, Florida 33602

Robert B. Furlough
Division of Mental Health
200 E. Gaines Street
Tallahassee, Florida 32304

Olive Galloway
University of South Florida
3622 S. Coolidge
Tampa, Florida 33609

Hugh Gaston
3210 Old Dawson Road
Albany, Georgia 31701

Alden S. Gilmore
University of South Florida
SOC 345
Tampa, Florida 33620

Robert Giudice, D.S.C.
Podiatrist
118 SW. 4th Avenue
Gainesville, Florida 32601

Donald L. Granger
R.F.D. 2, Box 4368
Fort Pierce, Florida 33450

Dan L. Green
305 Adams Drive
Crestview, Florida 32536

Sarinthia A. Gushanas
1920 Montmarte
Jacksonville, Florida 32210

Jack Hardy
Masonic Home of Florida
125-32nd Avenue Northeast
St. Petersburg, Florida 33704

Betty J. Heinemann
Route 1, Box 144
Williston, Florida 32696

Health Care Services for the Aged

Mrs. Ardith W. Highleyman
601 North Newman Street
Jacksonville, Florida 32202

Lucille W. Hill
8104 26th Avenue North
St. Petersburg, Florida 33710

Selden G. Hill
1103 Emeralda Drive
Orlando, Florida 32808

Miss Mary Eva Hite
Batesburg, South Carolina 29006

Edgar W. Homrighausen, D.D.
19301 SW. 87th Avenue
Miami, Florida 33157

L. F. Howbert
2208 SE. Lake Weir Road
Ocala, Florida 32670

James M. Hull
1071 S. Edgewood Avenue
Jacksonville, Florida 32205

Dr. George B. Hurff
Professor of Economics
342 Matherly Hall
University of Florida
Gainesville, Florida 32601

Mrs. Margaret A. Jacks
2818 Lydia Street
Jacksonville, Florida 32205

E. Russell Jackson
Florida Division of Health
P.O. Box 210
Jacksonville, Florida 32201

Floyd R. Jaggears
1945 Shady Oaks Drive
Tallahassee, Florida 32301

Miss Alice C. Jantzen
Professor of Occupational Therapy
A94 Teaching Hospital and Clinics
University of Florida
Gainesville, Florida 32601

Mrs. Ann Jenkins
1560 Lancaster Terrace
Jacksonville, Florida 32204

Mary Kay Jernigan
881 Peachtree Street Northeast
(Room 224)
Atlanta, Georgia 30309

Oliver Jernigan
University of South Florida
Tampa, Florida 33609

Collus O. Johnson
Georgia Gerontology Society, Inc.
DOCE, West Georgia College
Carrollton, Georgia 30117

Mary Johnson
Winter Park Towers
1111 South Lakemont Avenue
Winter Park, Florida 32789

Mrs. Hazel B. Johnwick
1710 NW. 16th Terrace
Gainesville, Florida 32601

Dorothy Jones
2020 N. Atlantic
Cocoa Beach, Florida 32931

Miss Elise C. Jones
Research Associate
221 Matherly Hall
University of Florida
Gainesville, Florida 32601

Helen D. Kaechele
1110 Alabama Drive
Winter Park, Florida 32787

George W. Karelas, M.D.
The Medical Rotunda
Newberry, Florida 32669

Alfred J. Karniewicz
3305 Korina Lane
Tampa, Florida 33618

Paul E. Kimberly, D.O.
4700 9th Avenue, North
St. Petersburg, Florida 33713

viii

Mrs. Paul E. Kimberly
4700 9th Avenue, North
St. Petersburg, Florida 33713

Victor King
1034 Dunraven Drive
Winter Park, Florida 32789

Sigmon S. Klein
420 Lincoln Road
Miami Beach, Florida 33139

Marjorie Knapp
Box 210
Jacksonville, Florida 32201

Sidney Knight
23 NW. 20th Drive—Apt. 4
Gainesville, Florida 32601

Lois N. Knowles
Assistant Dean
College of Nursing
University of Florida
Gainesville, Florida 32601

Thelma C. Langley
1108 Oxford Road
Atlanta, Georgia, 30306

Mrs. Grace Lanning
2828 Central Avenue
St. Petersburg, Florida 33712

Robert F. Lanzillotti
Dean and Professor
College of Business Administration
University of Florida
Gainesville, Florida 32601

Joseph H. Lavoie
4300 Alton Road
Miami Beach, Florida 33140

Homer Lawrence, Ed. D.
143 Sweetbay Drive
Jackson, Tennessee 38301

Mrs. Frank Lee
6021 SW. 13th Street
Gainesville, Florida 32601

Gerald R. Leslie
Professor of Sociology
308 Peabody Hall
University of Florida
Gainesville, Florida 32601

Aaron Lipman
University of Miami
8798 SW. 84th Street
Coral Gables, Florida 33124

Dorothy McCamman
Consultant
Group Health Association of America
  Incorporated
Washington, D.C.

Mary Lou McEver
3815 NW. 14th Place
Gainesville, Florida 32601

Helen M. McIntyre
2594 Columbus Way South
St. Petersburg, Florida 33712

Ira H. Mackie
2034 Ernest Street
Jacksonville, Florida 32204

Clifton W. McLoud
Florida Bureau on Aging
5410 Mariner
Tampa, Florida 33609

Wiley Mangum
Institute for Social Research
Florida State University
Tallahassee, Florida 32306

W. G. Martin
245 Beachview Drive
Fort Walton Beach, Florida 32548

Darrel J. Mase
Dean and Professor
College of Health Related Professions
University of Florida
Gainesville, Florida 32601

Olin J. Mason
Box 273
Sebring, Florida 33870

Glen Mauzy
P.O. Box 10155
Tampa, Florida 33602

Dr. Louis H. Meeth
901 Canterbury Road
Clearwater, Florida 33516

Louis A. Melsheimer
156 23rd Avenue
St. Petersburg, Florida 33704

Mrs. Sally H. Miller
1200 45th Street
West Palm Beach, Florida 33407

Grace D. Monk
210 Highland Drive
Americus, Georgia 31709

Bernice L. Morris
4606 Longfellow Ave.
Tampa, Florida 33609

Captain Danny R. Morrow
505 North Main Street
Jacksonville, Florida 32202

Dorothy V. Moses
6311 Lake Alamor
San Diego, California 92119

Blanche A. Murray
601 North Newnan Street
Jacksonville, Florida 32202

M. N. Newquist, M.D.
15 Hibiscus Road
Clearwater, Florida 33516

Daniel J. Novack
8400 NW. 25th Avenue
Miami, Florida 33147

Nancy A. Odell
310 Circle Drive
DeFuniak Springs, Florida 32433

Betty S. Orsini
501 79th Street South
St. Petersburg, Florida 33707

Lou O'Steen
307 North Ashley Drive
Tampa, Florida 33602

Carter C. Osterbind
Research Professor
College of Business Administration
221 Matherly Hall
University of Florida
Gainesville, Florida 32601

Richard D. Palmer
Educational Coordinator
Division of Continuing Education
University of Florida
Gainesville, Florida 32601

Robert E. Palmer
College of Education
University of South Florida
Tampa, Florida 33620

Harold Parker
881 Peachtree Street
Atlanta, Georgia 30309

Robert L. Parry
2001 18th Street West
Bradenton, Florida 33505

Col. Albert W. Paul
5016 Leona Street
St. Petersburg, Florida 33609

Maurice Pearlstein
7905 East Drive
North Bay Village, Florida 33141

Lloyd C. Peeples
3626 Sedgewick
Orlando, Florida 32806

Mrs. Fern M. Pence
P.O. Box 2050
Jacksonville, Florida 32203

Jean Jones Perdue, M.D.
6421 North Bay Road
Miami Beach, Florida 33141

Derek L. Phillips
Associate Professor of Sociology
Graduate School of Arts and Sciences
New York University
New York, New York

Claire Miller Pitzke
343 West 63rd Street
Jacksonville, Florida 32208

J. A. Powell
5016 Leona Street
Tampa, Florida 33609

Charles W. Pruitt
256 East Church Street
Jacksonville, Florida 32202

Lawrence Rackow
1436 Cheshire Road
Jacksonville, Florida 32207

John Rawls
4215 Granada Street
Tampa, Florida 33609

M. F. Reager
838 NE. Conway
Port Charlotte, Florida 33950

Lisa Renner
625 NW. 36th Avenue
Gainesville, Florida 32601

Dorothy P. Rice
Chief, Health Insurance Research
   Branch
Social Security Administration
United States Department, Health,
   Education, and Welfare
Washington, D.C.

Henry E. Richards
Caldwell Building
Tallahassee, Florida 32304

William W. Roberts
706 South Ride
Tallahassee, Florida 32303

Mrs. Rowena E. Rogers
151 East Minnehaha Avenue
Clermont, Florida 32711

Anna M. Russell
Kokeena Gates
Jacksonville, Florida 32207

Janet Ryan
1116 NW. 76th Avenue
Hollywood, Florida 33024

Warren N. Samples
P.O. Box 4466
Jacksonville, Florida 32201

Hyman K. Schonfeld
Associate Professor of Public Health
Department of Epidemiology and
   Public Health
Yale University
New Haven, Connecticutt 06520

Ben J. Schultz
Wesley Manor
Jacksonville, Florida 32223

Audrey S. Schumacher
Professor of Psychology
109 Building F
University of Florida
Gainesville, Florida 32601

Reverend B. F. Schumacher
19301 SW. 87th Avenue
Miami, Florida 33157

Elmer H. Shafer
401 South Prospect
Clearwater, Florida 33516

Power H. Sharretts
409 East Broward
Fort Lauderdale, Florida 33301

F. M. Shenk
3039 Samara Drive
Tampa, Florida 33618

Dr. Lester Sielski
School of Social Welfare
Florida State University
Tallahassee, Florida 32306

Edna M. Smiley
Box 324
Crescent City, Florida 32012

Health Care Services for the Aged

Rear Admiral Allen Smith, Jr.
43 Manor Drive
Pensacola, Florida 32507

Quentin M. Smith
College of Dentistry
University of Florida
Gainesville, Florida 32601

Anne R. Somers
Research Associate
Industrial Relations Section
Princeton University
Princeton, New Jersey 08540

Herman M. Somers
Professor of Politics and Public Affairs
Princeton University
Princeton, New Jersey 08540

Melton Spear
Older American Service Division
Administration on Aging
United States Department of Health,
    Education, and Welfare
Washington, D.C.

Mildred A. Sterling
1156 Westlawn Drive
Jacksonville, Florida 32211

Mrs. Grace Stewart
227 Park Street
Jacksonville, Florida 32204

Rita Storz
601 North Newman
Jacksonville, Florida 32202

Carol E. Taylor
Research Associate in Nursing
University of Florida
Gainesville, Florida 32601

R. E. Timberlake, Jr.
116 Jones Street
Raleigh, North Carolina 27601

Donald W. Trent
50 7th Street
Atlanta, Georgia 30308

Roger Turenne
3130 Santa Monica Drive
Decatur, Georgia 33032

Gail Valentine
1501 North Federal Highway
Lake Worth, Florida 33460

Al Volker
10625 SW. 82nd Avenue
Miami, Florida 33156

Constance G. Walker
5410 Mariner
Tampa, Florida 33609

Irving L. Webber
Professor of Sociology
450 College Library
University of Florida
Gainesville, Florida 32601

Harold N. Webster
3726 NE. 4th Street
Ocala, Florida 32670

Darlene Wheeler
256 East Church Street
Jacksonville, Florida 32202

Mrs. Mildred Whitlock
4300 Alton Road
Miami Beach, Florida 33140

Al Wilson
University of South Florida
Tampa, Florida 33610

Dr. Merrill Wise, Jr.
Tennessee Commission on Aging
Jackson, Tennessee 38301

Edwin L. Wood
P.O. Box 466
Roanoke, Virginia 24018

Mae S. Woodford
Route 1, Box 139
Hernando, Florida 32642

Robert P. Wray
Athens, Georgia 30601

Rex Wright
1713 Sherwood
Tallahassee, Florida 32303

Frank C. Wutz
201 Curtiss Parkway
Miami Springs, Florida 33166

Grant Youmans
University of Kentucky
Lexington, Kentucky 40506

George Young
1340 West 8th Street
Riviera Beach, Florida 33404

Delores Zeigler
South Carolina State Board of Health
Columbia, South Carolina

Cooperating Agencies

Administration on Aging, HEW, Washington, D.C.

Administration on Aging, HEW, Region IV, Atlanta

Adult and Veteran Section, Florida Department of Education

Alabama Commission on Aging

Altrusa International, Inc.

American Association of Retired Persons

American Cancer Society, Florida Division, Inc.

American Nursing Home Association

American Physical Therapy Association, Florida Chapter

Arkansas Office on Aging

Council on Gerontology, University of Georgia

Division of Community Hospitals and Medical Facilities, Board of Commissioners of State Institutions, Tallahassee, Florida

Division of Vocational Rehabilitation, Mississippi

Douglas Gardens, Jewish Home for the Aged of Greater Miami

Economic Development Division, U.S. Department of Agriculture

Florida Academy of Sciences

Florida Agricultural Extension Service, University of Florida

Florida Association of Homes for the Aging

Florida Association for Mental Health

Florida Association of Sheltered Workshops

Florida Bureau of Alcoholic Rehabilitation

Florida Bureau on Aging

Florida Conference of Social Welfare

Florida Council for the Blind

Florida Council of Churches

Florida Council on Aging

Florida Department of Education

Florida Department of Health and Rehabilitative Services

Florida Division of Family Services

Florida Division of Health

Florida Division of Labor, Bureau of Employment Services

Florida Division of Mental Health

Florida Division of Veterans Affairs

Florida Division of Vocational Rehabilitation

Health Care Services for the Aged

Florida Federation of Senior Clubs, Inc.

Florida Heart Association, Inc.

Florida Hospital Association

Florida Joint Council on Health of the Aging

Florida League for Nursing, Inc.

Florida Library Association

Florida Nurses Association

Florida Nursing Home Association

Florida Occupational Therapy Association

Florida Osteopathic Medical Association

Florida Rehabilitation Association

Florida Retired Teachers Association

Florida Society of Medical Technologists

Florida Speech and Hearing Association

Florida State Chamber of Commerce

Florida State Dental Association

Georgia Gerontology Society, Inc.

Gerontology Branch, Public Health Service, HEW, Atlanta, Georgia

Gerontological Society, Inc.

Governor's Committee on Aging, Texas

Hospitality House, AARP, St. Petersburg, Florida

Institute for Human Adjustment, Division of Gerontology, University of Michigan

Louisiana Commission on Aging

Lutheran Senior Citizens' Foundation, Inc., Miami

Maryland Commission on Aging

Memorial Home Community, Penney Farms, Florida

Model Cities Administration, DHUD, Atlanta

Mound Park Hospital Foundation, Inc., St. Petersburg, Florida

National Council on the Aging

National Retired Teachers Association

National Retired Teachers Association, Florida Division

Office of Economic Opportunity, Atlanta, Ga.

Orange County Citizens Advisory Council on Aging, Inc.

Pinellas County Health Department

Presbyterian Homes of the Synod of Florida

Retired Citizens Association of Florida, Inc.

River Garden, Hebrew Home for the Aged, Jacksonville, Florida

Salhaven—UIU Gerontological Village, Jupiter, Florida

Senior Citizen Services of Metropolitan Atlanta, Inc.

State Commission on Aging, Georgia

South Carolina Interagency Council on Aging

Tennessee Commission on Aging

The Senior Service Foundation (Miami, Florida)

William Crane Gray Inn for Older People, Davenport, Florida

Contents

xviii

Preface

by Carter C. Osterbind

A BROAD PROGRAM is being sponsored by the federal government to bring about improvements in health services in the United States. In 1968 the National Center for Health Services Research and Development was established in the United States Department of Health, Education, and Welfare. The purpose of the center is to serve as the focal point for health services research and development. It provides financial support and leadership in a national program of research, development, demonstration, and training projects addressed to major problems in the availability, organization, distribution, utilization, quality, and financing of health services, facilities, and technical equipment. Through the center's program it is hoped that innovations and improvements will be developed in organizing, delivering, and financing health services. The broadness of the program and the many types of research to which it gives attention indicate the complexity of the health care problem. The Nineteenth Annual Southern Conference on Gerontology has directed its program to the problems and prospects in effective use of resources in the health care of older people. In doing so the objective was not to thoroughly cover this broad subject but rather to direct attention to some continuing critical problems and to types of research and related efforts in the health care field that require public attention.

The program, while selective, covers a variety of topics. It touches on the need to develop measures against which programs may be evaluated; to focus on the rising cost of medical care; to envision an appropriate delivery structure both as it relates to the hospital, to ancillary services, and to related long-term care facilities; to obtain measures of the need for manpower and related inputs in relation to standards for planning good medical care; to relate the impact of chronic diseases on economic productivity; to discern the effective roles of health personnel; and to assess the attributes of the receivers of health care services that may influence their use of such services. The diversity of these topics suggests the variety of research needed to provide information on which to base plans to bring about the more effective use of resources in the health care field.

The speakers are from many parts of the country and we appreciate their willingness to participate. Over the years the conference has been supported by many individuals and groups in Florida, in the southeast, and in the nation. We are glad to have three supporting groups meeting here at this time: The Fifth Annual Clinical Session on Gerontological and Geriatric Nursing; the Florida Bureau on Aging; and the Florida Council on Aging. All three of these groups participated in the program plans for the conference and assisted in various other ways.

Also lending continuing support to the conference are the cooperating agencies representing units of federal and state governments and private organizations. We are pleased that there were a number of representatives of various state commissions on aging who participated in the conference. To all of these individuals and groups we are indebted for their contributions.

In addition to those whose papers are contained in the proceedings, the Council of the Institute of Gerontology expresses its appreciation to Mr. Robert Palmer, past President of the Florida Council on Aging; Dr. Jean Perdue, President of the Florida Council on Aging; Dr. Robert F. Lanzillotti, Dean of the College of Business Administration; Dr. John M. Champion, Professor of Health and Hospital Administration; Dr. Irving L. Webber, Professor of Sociology; Dr. George B. Hurff, Professor of Economics; and Mr. C. W. McLoud, Chief, Florida Bureau on Aging. Each of these individuals chaired conference sessions, led discussion groups or in other ways participated in the program. The council also expresses its appreciation to Mrs. Helen Kaechele and her co-workers from the Florida Council on Aging for their services as hostesses.

Social Indicators to Measure the Needs of Older People

by MEL SPEAR

THE TERM "social indicator" is quite new. *Social Indicators*, edited by Raymond A. Bauer and published in 1965, stirred initial interest in this area. This collection of thoughts on the need for adequate measures of social conditions was a by-product of an assignment to assess the impact of the space program on American life. The authors readily came to the conclusion that adequate tools for describing the American society were not available and that there was even less ability to assess the impact upon it of the space program. To quote them: "Though our interest originated with the problem of detecting the impact of the space program, the problem of measuring the impact of a single program could not be dealt with except in the context of the entire set of social indicators used in our society."[1] In 1967, the American Academy of Political and Social Science published *Social Goals and Indicators for American Society*. Early in 1969, the Department of Health, Education, and Welfare, published *Toward a Social Report*. Each of these papers explores such topics as health, crime, poverty, and expresses the need for, as well as the problems in, the development of social indicators. All of these efforts are exploratory and pose intriguing problems in constructing indicators to measure social conditions.

1. (Cambridge, Mass.: Massachusetts Institute of Technology), p. 1.

The history and development of precise indices is very recent. Up to the beginning of the Second World War, all quantitative economic and financial data, and all the related statistical techniques and methods which were concurrently developed, took the form either of indices of price levels, productive activity and employment, or of trends in financial activity. It was only during the Second World War and immediately after it that there was a realization that these aggregated data could be of immediate practical use and interest to government authorities, to large enterprises, to labor organizations, and to all other similar decision-making bodies. Statisticians also became convinced that only a system of interlocking aggregates in an articulated framework could disclose any coherence or incoherence in the data collected from different and varied sources. It could, at the same time, bring into light the areas of ignorance and the missing links of data and information.

Three methodological systems were soon developed. One system attempts primarily to measure the national income, final product, consumption, and accumulation of capital. The second system is largely devoted to the presentation of the inter-industrial process of production and the movement of commodities. The main role of the third system is to show how production processes, consumption, and investment are currently financed. The common denominator of these three systems is that they all deal with the flowing process of economic and financial activities. They describe the flow of the contributions of labor to production and the reverse flow of income labor receives from productive enterprises; they show the flow of intermediate commodities between the various branches of national industry and the flow of finished goods to consumers. Such systems also display the circular financial flows which permit real goods and services to flow between the various large segments of the economy.

Each of the above systems has been independently constructed, mainly during the last three decades, and has been put into extensive practical and theoretical use, particularly in the industrially developed countries of the Western world. These methodological sets of accounts have become commonly known as social accounting systems.

Today, there are many indicators in use. They are particularly prevalent in the areas where quantitative data is readily available and where the units of measurement stem from a common base, such as dollars. The further removed from these conditions, the less common the use of indicators will be. Thus, while the use of indicators is very common in the area of economics, they are less common and largely nonexistent in the social areas. Some examples of indicators in different areas follow.

Economic indicators.—consumer price index (cost of living index), unemployment index, gross national product, interest rate (serves as an indicator in addition to its more obvious functional role), national debt, federal budget, balance of payments, gold reserves, corporation profits, inventory stockpiles, Dow Jones Industrial Average (as well as other similar stock market indicators), tax rates (also have an obvious functional role).

Physical environment indicators.—radition count (and other pollution indicators), normal temperatures, accumulated index of precipitation, degree days, required heating units, population density, pollen index, caloric intake.

National defense indicators.—nuclear submarine gap, overkill, missile gap, striking power, standing army, battle deaths, retaliation force.

Moral-psychological indicators.—FBI crime index, suicide rate, divorce rate, birth rate, illegitimate birth rate.

Health indicators.—death rate from cancer and infant mortality rate (and various other causes of death), life expectancy, work loss, rejection rate for draftees (physical causes), hospital admissions.

Educational indicators.—illiteracy rate (no longer common in this country), rejection rate for draftees (literacy), educational attainment test results.

Political activity indicators.—voter turnout, voter profiles, registered voters.

As more and more sophisticated methods come into practice, we are even beginning to see a new level of measurement emerging, called mood measurement. Since the mental and emotional disposition precedes the act, whether in sports, crime, business, or any other human endeavor, thousands of individuals are engaged every day in mood measurement.

Most of these researchers have little to do with mental health clinics; their interest in moods is not psychiatric but financial, for it has been found that the human mood can effect the economy more strongly than a presidential act.

Among the measurements used in arriving at economic conclusions are these: Index of Consumer Sentiment, maintained by the Survey Research Center at the University of Michigan; Sales Optimism Index, maintained by Dun and Bradstreet, (measures the per cent of businessmen expecting sales gains, minus those expecting decreases); Help Wanted Advertising Index, a production of the National Industrial Conference Board (a measurement of how actively employers are seeking workers); Purchasing agent polls; and Investor Confidence Index.

Not being a researcher myself nor directly engaged in this exploratory effort, I must disclaim attributes of expertise. What I prefer to present to you, is the effort of the Administration on Aging to construct a systematic system for measuring the social condition of the aged. The Administration on Aging has awarded a three-year grant for research by the American Rehabilitation Foundation for "A Social Indicator System for the Aging." I am indebted to the American Rehabilitation Foundation for the technical aspects they have reported and described in their exploration of preliminary social indicator concepts. I draw heavily upon their work.

Before we get too far into the discussion let's define social indicator. A social indicator has been defined as a single number, empirically derived as a single number by a transformation of data related to a social condition. This number or social indicator relates to the social condition (or conditions) judged by society to be a significant contributor to individual or group well-being.

The first objective of the research is to design a system of social indicators to describe the status of older Americans. Another objective in the computation of social indicators for the aged is to use the system to give us a measure of national achievement toward the attainment of essential goals for older Americans. The resulting social indicators will be developed in time for, and in association with, planning being undertaken for the 1971 White House Conference on Aging.

It is anticipated that the indicators will provide those planning for and participating in the White House Conference with a clear picture of the status of older Americans. This is extremely important for two reasons: First, such a picture does not currently exist; and second, it is extremely helpful if not necessary for the development of a rational social policy.

The current situation is expressed in the following quote: ". . . social statistics, in their present form, rarely seem to tell us what we need to know for informed policy planning. . . . It is exceedingly difficult to construct an adequate picture of current changes . . . among different population groups . . . from the social statistics that are readily available. When trying to assess the requirements and preferences of distinct groups of people or to trace the impact of our present policies and programs, standard sources are scarcely illuminating. As a result, the sweep of our policy judgments about central issues is rarely inhibited by the burden of factual information. . . .

". . . The development of a set of social indicators and the consequent improvement of our empiric information .can contribute greatly . . . to more rational social policy."[2]

I do not mean to imply that our currently available statistics are not valuable. As Shakespeare has remarked, "the fault, dear Brutus, lies in us." Many stories circulate about the statisticians delight, the average man. It is said that this fractional being lives somewhere in the middle area of the country with .864 of a wife who has borne him 2.013 children. Occasionally, like the headless horror of Irving's stories, he terrorizes the countryside by driving at night in his 1.356 of an automobile, colliding with some other object, causing .0019 of an accident and getting himself .000146 killed. These figures are not accurate, but they give you some idea of how these daily lottery figures can be played for the percentages.

Since Americans are convinced of the mathematical certainty of modern life, we might speculate on how to conduct ourselves in the light of present statistics. For instance, though travel on the highways is extremely hazardous, experts say that more accidents occur in the home. Thus, to stay alive longer, the odds are that

2. Doris B. Holleb, "Social Statistics for Social Policy," *Planning 1968*, pp. 80, 85.

you should stay away from home. From a study of life-expectancy tables, for those who want to live long, we should by comparison of various indicators—pollution, DDT levels, radiation levels, urban impact—decide to move, perhaps to the Arizona desert. Each year we could get the annual indicator-supplement and move to a new and safer location according to the latest charts. I suppose if you are so inclined, you might consider such an inane proposal. But don't forget, if you follow this advice you might be helping to change these statistics; and furthermore, you might also get so worn down from moving that your fatigue would lead you to ill-ness and then to such debilitation that you might wish you were dead.

It is envisioned that the indicators constructed by the study will be limited specifically to the provision of a clear picture of social conditions and will *not*, at this time, assign normative values to those social indicators selected. There are two basic areas that are currently under review: (1) the concept itself as it pertains to a systematic description of social conditions of the aged; and (2) the selection of relevant social conditions.

The study team, in its first phase of operations, undertook an extensive review of the literature available on the subject. While a great deal has not been published on this subject, there is a lack of consistent terminology—social indicators, social statistics, social ac-counting—each assigned different meanings by its authors. The re-search team has met with others in the field, both researchers and gerontological practitioners. They have reviewed many potential sources of data for computing social indicators.

A significant concept emerges in the definitions separating a social condition and a social action. A condition is the actual exist-ence or observable state of an individual's or group's situation. An action is something undertaken that relates to the condition. Thus, the level of health of older Americans is their social condition. The action is the amount of resources being spent for Medicare. As so-cial indicators are expressed in numerical quantities, the social con-dition may be described in a figure which increases or decreases. We then have some index expressed as a social indicator of well-being. The social conditions may be determined on the observa-tions gathered from competent observers. It may also include the first-hand knowledge from the aged person's response to questions either in an interview or by a self-completed questionnaire.

By monitoring conditions through observation and transforming these fundamental observations into a concise quantitative report, we obtain a clear picture of existing social conditions.

This, primarily, is the function of social indicators. For example, we could provide a picture of the income status of older Americans by computing indicators on a periodic basis to show how their income changes over time as contrasted to their basic needs and how their status compares to those of other age populations. From such comparisons a more explicit statement of national goals may be possible, and the report would provide a means of measuring progress toward those goals.

SELECTING RELEVANT SOCIAL CONDITIONS

One of the more difficult aspects of this study is the value judgments necessary to select the relevant social conditions. We are far from a consensus on which social conditions are relevant. A second value judgment must be made in defining each condition after it has been selected. For example, after health has been selected as a relevant social condition, additional judgments are required to obtain the explicit definition of "observation of states" that are included. Are chronic health problems included along with acute episodes of illness? Are headaches, colds or arthritis included among other major health problems as are heart conditions or high blood pressure? And what about the relative worth of each state? In the definition of a social indicator, judgments about the *relative value* of the different states must be explicitly stated. The assignment of a relative value, or relative worth or non-worth, must be made between a chronic condition such as a heart condition on one hand and an acute condition such as a broken hip. These value judgments are necessary in order to make an aggregation possible.

It is interesting to compare the problems experienced by others and the value judgments that have been exercised in construction of indicators. The FBI crime index is fairly well-known and is quite frequently published in the nation's newspapers as are other indicators—unemployment index, cost of living, etc. Crime was selected

7

as a relevant social condition from among *all* social conditions. This was a value judgment by the FBI. Then, a set of crimes which would be included in the index were selected. Seven crimes— homicide, rape, aggravated assault, robbery, burglary, larceny, and auto theft—were included, all others excluded including kidnapping and arson. Each crime was considered equal. Thus, only the total number of crimes affect the numerical quantity of the index. The originators of the crime index made a value judgment and defined the aggregation problem by allowing the crime index to reflect that one murder is equal to one auto theft or one robbery.

The study team suggests, tentatively, that there are five major relevant social conditions currently defined: income; health; shelter; socialization; and attitudes or life satisfaction. (These major categories will be broken down into finer categories as the study progresses.)

It is important not only to measure the social conditions of the aged, but also to determine the attitude of the aged toward these conditions. To undertake social actions that will improve the social conditions of the aged, from the viewpoint of the aged, it will be necessary to know how the aged themselves feel about their life and what expectations they have. The attitudes of other classes of people toward the elderly and their problems may also be extremely important in improving social conditions for the aged.

The technical aspects of the construction of a system, obtaining data, assigning weighted values and relative weights to some normative scale, I am certain, will be done in due time.

What concerns me is the urgency with which we must focus on needs in order that we may achieve the goals we envision on behalf of the elderly. I represent a program, administered by fifty state agencies implementing the Older Americans Act, that in a very brief period of time has shown extremely successful program accomplishments. Each state has developed a state agency focused primarily on aging, which has become a focal point in state government for planning and coordination, for evaluation of resource allocation, and for leadership and advocacy on behalf of the aged. More than 1,200 community projects have been funded since passage of the Older Americans Act.

There are still wide gaps in many communities in effective delivery of services for the elderly even though many hundreds of communities and neighborhoods have initiated effective programs for the elderly.

Changes in the age structure of society, accompanied by changes that are so rapidly taking place, have set the stage for the evolution of a national aging policy.[3]

A SOCIAL POLICY ON AGING

Since social indicators ultimately are dependent upon a consensus of social policy positions, it is appropriate, therefore, that we turn our attention to the development of a social policy on aging. We are not only dependent upon the competent observation and the data that identifies the needs, but we must also be able to interpret the sense of society at a given time, and translate that sensitivity through what is called "the art of politics" into legislative mandates, into appropriate and needed funding, and into adequate and effective administrative, operative mechanisms.

The difficulty with respect to meeting the needs of the aging lies in the fact that there are extremely limited areas in which explicit social policy has been evidenced. Two areas come readily to mind. In income maintenance the concepts of social insurance and public assistance for the aged are not controversial. While adequacy remains at low levels, and is often in controversy, a minimal floor of income support for the aged cannot be denied. Similarly, by enactment of the 1965 amendments to the Social Security Act—Medicare and Medicaid—Congress has given tangible expression to health care as a basic human right. The means for the purchase of health care, in the hands of the aged and the poor, and such purchase at the place of their own choosing and choice, gives tacit acknowledgment that the doctrine of "Separate but Equal" is no more valid in the health field than it is for the educational system.

However, when we begin to move into other areas of social need which require government action, a value system more related to the frontier society and to the concepts of the Elizabethan

3. John C. McKinney and Frank T. deVyver, *Aging and Social Policy* (New York: Appleton-Century-Crofts, 1966).

9

Poor Laws and to the Puritan value of productive labor begins to manifest itself. The dominant feature of this value system is the importance it assigns to the independence of the American citizen coupled with the idea that the least government is the best government. This is an ethic highly valued. Yet one must wonder whether it tends toward tunnel vision particularly when it is related to the dependent status of the aged and the necessity for a governmental role in developing a support system for the poor, the frail, and disabled aged as well as for their retirement that stretches on without blessing. Even the efforts of the elderly to maintain that desired independence is often met with indifference and hostility by key decision-makers.

It is often argued that the poor are to blame for their own circumstances and should be expected to lift themselves from poverty. The simple fact is that most poor remain poor because access to income through work is currently beyond their reach.[4] The aged possess limited earning potential. Old age is usually a period of non-employment and society neither expects nor assists the aged to work. They generally are expected to live on pensions, savings, social security benefits, public assistance grants. Too frequently savings and pensions deemed adequate at an earlier time become insufficient as inflation raises the cost of living. Millions of hardworking Americans, accustomed all their lives to paying their way, find themselves becoming unalterably and unavoidably poor in old age.

. In 1966 more than six million aged persons and their dependents were in poverty. Opportunities for the aged poor to make any improvement in their own lives are remote and unrealistic. Only public programs can make a difference in their incomes.

To quote from the Income Maintenance Programs Report *Poverty Amid Plenty*: "Absolute poverty must be ended soon in the U.S. By its very existence, absolute poverty condemns some citizens to death or lives of misery. This should not be tolerated amidst the vast wealth of our Nation."[5]

As a nation we are only now coming to a realization that the

4. *Poverty Amid Plenty: The American Paradox,* report of the President's Commission on Income Maintenance Programs, 1969.
5. *Ibid.,* p. 41.

financing of health service involves more than a fiscal response to what has been categorized as an aggregation of a series of purely private transactions.

We have federal programs such as Medicaid, Medicare, and others which finance the purchase of personal health services, but we have yet to obtain out of this the kind of health care delivery system that improves the nation's health or has provided the quality care we are capable of producing for more and better health care.

We need more concrete measures undertaken to encourage the use of desirable alternatives to inpatient hospital care and nursing home care services. We need to give priority to development of organized primary health care services in neighborhoods; development of services such as home health care programs; social and other outreach services which are an integral aspect of appropriate utilization of services; the development of ways to link and relate new and existing health services with each other aiming toward comprehensive health care systems in communities.[6]

We must move beyond simplistic response in meeting basic needs and cope with those problems that lie beyond and below the surface of our awareness. We must not become so brutalized, so unfeeling and insensitive, that only individual comfort and well-being are pitted against the reality of poverty, illness, and prejudice.

It is infinitely complicated to reason about an ideal society. Society is so complex that few men, or none at all, could judge a blueprint for social engineering on the grand scale.

Even the survival of the human community on earth may already be a utopian ideal. For its realization, we have little experience, tools, training, or organization. We lack even the will to proceed with the long-range planning needed, community, national, and global, to meet tomorrow's resolutions of hunger and unfulfilled expectations or today's reality of poverty and disease. Martin Luther King said at the Washington Cathedral, shortly before he died, "We are sleeping through a revolution."

The point I want to emphasize in closing is that it is not enough

6. Recommendations of the Task Force on Medicaid and Related Programs, United States Department of Health, Education, and Welfare, November, 1969.

that we know what needs to be done, but it is important and necessary to back the knowledge we have with action.

Aristotle tells of an old citizen of Athens who attended the Olympic games at the Coliseum. He went first to the section occupied by the Athenians. No one rose from the crowded section to offer him a seat. When he went to the Spartan section several youths leaped to their feet, offering him their place. The Athenians noticing that the old man finally had a seat jumped to their feet and cheered. The old man then, with tears in his eyes said, "All the Athenians know what is right, but only the Spartans practice it."

Inflation in Medical Care Costs

by HERMAN SOMERS

I CONFESS that I was initially reluctant when the chairman of this conference invited me to discuss the assigned subject. It seemed that an audience like this, interested in medical care, would find inflation and high costs tired subjects, painfully familiar, and old hat.

Second thoughts, however, led me to believe that this itself might dictate the desirability of accenting this subject once again, because there is a social danger of sheer accustomization to inflation leading to a mood of resigned acceptance. The problem is too important to allow us the luxury of lethargy or to allow us to confuse the long repetitive occurrence with inevitability. Inflation and costs are matters that can be acted upon; they are controllable.

Traditionally, interest in costs of health care has focused upon the extent that costs might signify significant barriers to essential care. The existence of such barriers is, of course, a vital matter. But cost experience can tell us a great deal more. Costs (meaning the product of prices and utilization) are not independent or isolated phenomena. If viewed analytically, cost data can serve as essential indicators respecting all significant issues in the organization, financing, and delivery of health care.

When prices evidence highly unusual or inconsistent patterns, it is usually a sign of maladjustment between supply and demand.

13

Such maladjustment may merely represent a temporary transitional period toward a changed level of stability or it may bespeak more profound structural inadequacies which may not be self-correcting. Cost data will not in themselves reveal all the complex causes, and surely not the solutions of the maladjustment. But if their signals are properly observed, they can tell us when and where there is trouble that needs attending.

Our recent history has, in fact, moved in accordance with such a pattern. Public concern was first expressed in reaction to the staggering inflation of costs, an inflation unmatched in intensity and duration. It was this experience, and its attendant resentments, that focused an unprecedented spotlight on the health care industry. Once the glare began to penetrate the many recesses of this complex field, it appeared to reveal an array of alleged difficulties: a delivery system (or non-system as it is often called) fraught with inefficiency, obsolete arrangements, inequities, and waste—all increasingly criticized by professionals as well as laymen, but apparently intractable to quick or obvious reform.

Indicative of the heights of public policy to which the broad issue has advanced, on July 10, 1969, the President of the United States forecast over national television a "massive crisis" in health care within the next two or three years unless prompt action was taken. The occasion was his receipt of a White House report from the Secretary of the Department of Health, Education, and Welfare and the Assistant Secretary for Health and Scientific Affairs which stated, "This nation is faced with a breakdown in the delivery of health care unless immediate concerted action is taken by Government and the private sector."

The two phenomena—high costs and a disjointed or inadequate delivery system—nurture one another. The now common awareness of the relationship has made it clear that the problem will not be met successfully by exclusive dependence on arbitrary price fixing, cost ceilings, or any instruments directed solely to dollar controls, although such devices are not to be disregarded. Concern has now been drawn increasingly to the delivery system—its productivity, its adequacy, and effectiveness. This has enhanced quality consciousness and sensitivity to the wide variations in value of particular services.

14

The degree of effectiveness of the various elements in the organization and financing of health care find expression in the costs of service. The lively current examination of the system is simply a rational pursuit of the inevitable question: What are we getting for our money?

II

Now let us turn for a moment to a few of the basic facts. I hope you will bear with me through a few statistics.

Health care expenditures during the last fiscal year, 1969, continued their long rapid increase and reached over $60 billion. The growth in one year was almost $6½ billion, or 12 per cent, as it was also the year before. Per capita expenditures were four times as large as in fiscal year 1950, averaging an increase of 7.2 per cent each year.

Health expenditures have for a long time been rising faster than the nation's total output of goods and services. In fiscal year 1959, health outlays were 4.6 per cent of gross national product (GNP); by fiscal year 1969 they were 6.7 per cent. In nineteen years health care enlarged its share of GNP by 46 per cent. It must be remembered that the American economy has been expanding vigorously —eightfold in the last forty years. Even if health expenditures had remained on a constant relationship to the rest of the economy, they would have experienced a very substantial steady growth. But the rate at which health outlays have been outpacing GNP has been accelerating. Expenditures may approach 10 per cent by the end of this decade.

Many factors have contributed to this spectacular growth, including: a continuous enlargement of demand for health services, recently augmented by a sizeable expansion of government financing; new methods of financing, including the steady growth of health insurance; scientific and technological advances; and extraordinarily large increases in health care prices. These factors are, of course, interacting.

The various elements that constitute rising costs of health care are generally, in their most simplified form, classified into three broad categories: increases in total population; increased utilization of services (which includes increases in the level, or quality, of care); increased prices per unit of service.

All three have been moving up steadily, but at very different rates. Population has been growing, but, despite what we read about population pollution, not really at any overwhelming rate, only at about 1 per cent a year since 1965.

Per capita utilization has been growing much faster, averaging almost 3 per cent a year since 1950 and 4 per cent since 1960. This is not surprising and is easily explained by a number of social and economic phenomena, for example: large incomes; our changing demographic composition, such as the relative increase of women in the population, especially at older ages; urbanization of population; a shift in morbidity patterns from predominance of acute episodic illness to chronic, long-term ailments; increased public support of health care for the poor; growth of insurance and other third-party payments; the spectacular advances in medical technology which within this century converted medical care from a service of generally dubious effectiveness into a life-saving and life-enhancing essential.

Whatever the relative mix of these and other factors, Americans are conspicuously expressing their sense of need for more and improved health services, pressing hard against a supply that appears to have fallen far behind in quantity or structural adequacy or both.

Prominent among the frustrations that have accompanied growing demand is spiraling prices, the third broad category and by far the most important factor in explaining rising costs. In recent years, since 1965, medical care prices have been going up over 6 per cent each year and medical services (omitting drugs and supplies) over 7 per cent a year.

When these three factors are related to one another we find that for the nation as a whole the enormous increase in expenditures between 1950 and 1969, from $26 billion to $60 billion, was accounted for as follows:

Population increase explained 18 per cent. Increased services per capita (both quantity and quality) explained 35 per cent. Increased prices per unit of service accounted for 47 per cent, almost half.

Viewed from the perspective of the cost to the average individual—by eliminating the population growth factor and examining only the relative influence of the other two factors in additional expenditures for health care—the picture is even sharper. Per capita expenditures increased more than two and one-half times in that period, 1950 to 1969. About two-fifths, or 43 per cent, was due to additional use of services, and almost three-fifths was attributable to price change.

In short, of every added dollar spent by the average consumer, about 57 cents was washed away by higher prices. The additional dollar bought him 43 cents in additional real services.

Of course, prices have been going up everywhere. Price rise in the general economy has contributed to the inflation of medical prices. But the differential between general prices and health care price increases has been pronounced and persistent for more than two decades. Between 1946 and 1969 medical care prices advanced 155 per cent while the index of all prices advanced 88 per cent, an average annual increase of 4.7 per cent versus 2.8 per cent. By far the major influence was hospital daily service charges which increased 592 per cent, almost seven times as fast as all prices, and five times as fast as all services in the Consumer Price Index.

For years it was optimistically said that this was in large part a catching-up process, since medical prices had fallen behind other prices during the Great Depression and hospital wages were making up their lag behind other wage scales. After a reasonable period, the argument ran, we could expect a levelling out, and medical price increases would then be generally consistent with other price movements. The prediction has proved invalid. In recent years the differential has actually widened significantly. Last year, 1969, was an exception because general prices experienced an extraordinary inflation of 5.4 per cent. But even then medical care prices jumped more sharply, by 6.9 per cent.

The infusions of the large Medicare and Medicaid programs were undoubtedly partly responsible for the large increases since 1965, but they were only additional stimulants. The forces of inflationary momentum in the health economy appear more basic, and they long preceded the advent of the new programs. And they will outlast the current general inflation. Any validity that the

17

catching-up argument may have had in the past was surely outworn sometime ago.

III

The issue has, of course, reached dimensions to become a major national concern to all sectors of the economy. Such trends threaten the survival of the health insurance industry; they are an increasing burden upon large employers who pay the major share of health insurance premiums; they menace the hard fought for fringe benefits of labor unions; and they understandably are causing consternation in government circles.

Government at all levels spent almost $23 billion for medical care in fiscal year 1969, almost $18 billion of it for personal health services, the large bulk of which was provided by the federal government or stimulated by it under grant-in-aid programs. Government's relative share of all health care expenditures rose from 25 per cent to 38 per cent in three years. Much of this growth was the result of Medicare and Medicaid programs which expended $6.6 billion and $4.4 billion respectively in fiscal year 1969.

Cost inflation has been severely felt by government programs. Medicare and Medicaid are exceeding anticipated costs mainly due to greater price rises than seemed reasonable to allow for in earlier estimates. For the hospital insurance part of Medicare, Congress very early had to raise the projected long-term tax rate. The deductible and coinsurance paid by the patient have been increased twice within two years, a total of 30 per cent. Premiums for the supplementary medical insurance part of the program have also been increased twice, by a total of 77 per cent.

On the outlay side, Medicaid benefits have been cut back in a number of states, and Congress introduced restrictive limits on income levels for eligibility the year after the program went into effect. There is widely publicized dissatisfaction with the program for a variety of reasons, but much of it stems from soaring costs. In both programs, the administration has cut back its payment formulas to providers of care, and the latter have accused the government of welching on its obligations.

The outlook for the future is producing deep anxieties. Con-

18

sumer dissatisfactions are increasingly articulated and pressed upon both Congress and the administration. Projections of costs portend budgetary crises: If current trends are not abated, by 1975 medical expenditures could consume almost all of the Department of Health, Education, and Welfare's anticipated additional appropriations, thus depriving it of new initiatives in its wide range of other responsibilities and depriving it of priority judgments. Moreover, government finds that its great additional expenditures have not only failed to produce equitable utilization of health care resources by the whole population but that there has been small net gain. Secretary Robert Finch's and Doctor Roger O. Egeberg's report on the health of the nation's health care system spoke of the "crippling inflation in medical costs causing vast increases in government health expenditures for *little return,* raising private health insurance premiums and reducing the purchasing power of the health dollar of our citizens."

It has also become clear from government reports that its programs have failed to supply the medical needs of the poor and the black community. Public programs reach only a minority of the 40 million poor and near-poor, as officially defined, and there is considerable question about the extent of the need met even among those who are reached. Medicare is aimed at the aged and therefore does reach a group in which there is heavy concentration of poor and near-poor. Medicaid reached slightly more than 8 million people in 1969, about one-fifth of the poor and near-poor. But of the total Medicaid budget, about 46 per cent goes to the elderly, although they represent only about one-third of the recipients, presumably to cover gaps arising from the fact that Medicare pays for an average of only 45 per cent of health care expenditures of the aged. If the 2 million children who received services under Medicaid are added to the 400,000 under maternal and child health programs (disregarding overlaps) we find about 2.5 million children being aided compared to the 19 or 20 million children among the poor and near poor, about one child out of eight. The administration is sensitive to the social and political implications of these facts but faces the frustrations of high-flying costs.

All of this has resulted in substantial soul-searching in government, as it has in the insurance industry and among some providers of care. There is grave doubt being cast upon the allocation of government resources in this area; doubt, for example, about whether it is equitable or wise that about one-half of all government payments for personal health care is spent for the aged (only about one-eighth of government payments are for children under fifteen). There are more fundamental reservations about the division of expenditures between purchase of services and building an adequate supply capacity—a difficulty perceived to characterize the entire health care economy as well.

The rapid increase of costs has considerably curtailed leeway for allocation of more funds to augment supply under tight budgetary conditions, especially with rising resistance against pouring more money into a supply system that is widely believed to be using resources wastefully and at relatively low levels of productivity. There is growing sentiment that if new investment in supply is to be effective, it must be related to a redesigned delivery structure.

IV

As already indicated, prices appear to have been the most important element in cost rise in recent years, at least in relation to the two major services, hospital care and physicians' services. Explanations for the extraordinary price inflation are controversial. Different sectors of providers operate differently and are subject to different influences. The price behavior of the several sectors varies. Here we must confine our discussion to hospitals, the largest sector and the one in which price rise has been most pronounced.

Prominent among the more frequent justifications advanced for accelerated hospital costs are:

1. Medical and hospital technologies have been advancing at a phenomenal pace with commensurate demands on facilities, equipment, personnel, and services. Per capita, admittees use more services, such as diagnostic and therapeutic X-ray procedures, drugs, and laboratory services. There has been a growth in the range of services made available. For example, between 1963 and 1968 the proportion of community hospitals with intensive care services (including coronary care services) jumped from 18 per cent to 42 per

cent. The equipment for all such services grows more elaborate and costly, and its rate of obsolescence is more rapid.

2. The rise in labor costs is conspicuous. A by-product of advancing technology has been additional and more specialized personnel. Also, hospitals have been gradually catching up with long overdue improvements in wages and working conditions. Reduction in hours of work has caught up with other industries. A lag still exists in wages and the next few years will probably witness through law and bargaining an equalization between hospital and similar types of employment. Many hospital officials assert that when this occurs, hospital prices will stabilize in relation to other prices.

3. Hospitals have assumed increased functions in addition to direct patient care. Important among these is education. Despite the decline in hospital-based schools of nursing, they still account for about four-fifths of RN graduates, and the cost of these programs to the hospitals is rising. With federal subsidies for nurse education and the trend toward academic settings for such education, this burden should eventually decline, but it will be slow. Also, many hospitals have been adding full-time directors of medical education, an additional, although modest, factor in costs.

4. Hospital financing is increasingly coming through commercial borrowing, rather rare in the past. Interest charges, still a small part of total operating expenses, are nonetheless adding a new factor to hospital costs.

5. The common measure of hospital prices, the average per diem expense, is misleading. The factors in the numerator—total operating costs—have less and less relationship to the denominator —inpatient days. Hospitals increasingly engage in a variety of other services and activities; particularly there has been a rapid increase in outpatient services. The American Hospital Association has, therefore, recently developed a different denominator. It takes into account outpatient services by converting them into inpatient day equivalents, and deriving an "adjusted patient day" figure. This, of course, reduces the average per diem figure. However, studies indicate that when this adjustment is carried back in time the result has no significant effect upon price trends.

6. Another factor, perhaps overlapping point 1, is the changing

21

mix of patients. Patients with relatively serious illness, requiring the more complex and expensive procedures, represent an increasing proportion of the hospital population.

Critics of hospital costs do not find such explanations satisfying. As statements of fact, they are true, as far as they go. But they do not enlighten one on the extent of the price rise which each, or their aggregate, may explain. Nor do they indicate to what extent the factual developments are justifiable or necessary.

It cannot be questioned that there has been a great expansion of facilities, equipment, personnel, and services. But how much represents unnecessary duplication of facilities and equipment among several hospitals within the same community, because each hospital behaves as an autonomous unit rather than as part of a coordinated health care system? How much of the new equipment are prestige or convenience items?

How much of the mounting increase in ancillary services is simply a result of the spread of third-party payment which has reduced the physician's inhibitions to additional laboratory procedures or an additional day's stay in the hospital, and the individual consumer's resistance to higher costs, on which a normal market situation would place considerable reliance?

Has there been any attempt to measure the relative value to health care represented by new equipment and added services, or are "improved models" bought without such criteria because hospitals now have a virtual guarantee of repayment of all their costs from third-party payors? Has there been progress toward developing measures of cost-benefit relationships?

Payrolls have indeed increased and these are, of course, the major factor in hospital operating costs. But it is not true that payroll costs have advanced more rapidly than other costs in recent years. From 1960 to 1968, despite a substantial rise in personnel in relation to patient load, total expenses per patient day advanced more rapidly than payroll per patient day, 90 per cent against 82 per cent. Payrolls accounted for 62 per cent of total expenses in 1960 and 60 per cent in 1968.

Moreover, wage increases cannot be charged with the whole responsibility for payroll increases. The American Hospital Association attributes half of increased total expenditures for wages and salaries between 1963 and 1968 to additional employment. For many years hospitals have been steadily adding more and more personnel per patient. In the last five-year period alone, 1963–68, the number of employees per one thousand *adjusted* patient days increased 13 per cent.

The hospitals are accused of an insatiable capacity for absorbing more manpower, the only restraint being their availability. They had an alleged manpower crisis in 1950 when hospitals were employing 178 persons per 100 inpatients; now there are 272 employees per 100 inpatients—a striking increase of 53 per cent which cannot be fully explained by the growth of outpatient services—and a manpower crisis is even more loudly proclaimed. There are wide variations in the personnel-patient ratios among states, but there are no indications of any correlation with quality of care received or health results.

A major issue thus lies in the hospital's apparent failure or inability to employ new technology for productivity increases, which has characterized the rest of the American economy. Introduction of new equipment and procedures has been accompanied by more rather than less personnel. In fact, hospitals justify additional personnel by such developments. Increased wages in hospitals have not been matched by greater productivity, at least as this is now crudely measured.

Such data do not prove anything definitively, because quality —one element in productivity—has undoubtedly risen. But how much, or in what degree it is comparable to the rise in personnel or other resources, is not known. Nevertheless there appears some basis for a presumption that net productivity is falling or, at best, is static. One may concede that a labor-intensive personal service industry will have more difficulty improving productivity than will manufacturing firms. While precise parallels are never available, some other service industries—for example, financial institutions— have demonstrated that very significant gains can be made. Is it really impossible in hospitals? Or is there a lack in incentives, in skills, or in organizational structure that is inhibiting? Perhaps it is the eleemosynary tradition, or perhaps the persistent myths built around the special character of the service, that fosters the widely held notion that efficiency and concern for productivity are enemies of quality, a problem that prevails in education as well. The contrary is likely to be true. Effective quality control and cost control generally go hand in hand.

In a field notably lacking in satisfactory measures of unit costs, definitions of output, productivity, or effectiveness, neither side in the debate can prove its position conclusively. But the circumstantial evidence is great that the cost aberrations are an important symptom of basic organizational shortcomings. This is underpinned by increasing professional conviction that the delivery structure is obsolete and ineffective from a quality viewpoint as well. Thus, interestingly, those approaching the problem from the perspective of cost efficiency and those attacking it from a quality effectiveness view appear to have arrived at very similar sets of reform proposals. The two objectives are quite consonant.

The reform trends that are in motion (often promulgated by leaders in the hospital field) although multiple, can, like the criticisms, be said to fall into two broad classes: improvements in the delivery system, its organization and management; and changes in financing arrangements. The two overlap at many points. It is now better understood than it was only a decade ago that the character of financing influences the delivery system and vice versa.

It is not my assignment this morning, nor would I in any case have the time here, to speak about alterations due in the delivery system. The next paper on this program will be dealing with certain aspects of this problem. I must confine myself to calling attention to the fact that one cannot wisely appraise or correct cost problem without relation to the delivery structure.

V

In conclusion, I would like to spend a few moments to relate these issues to what I presume is your primary concern, the aged. I have already mentioned that about half of all government expenditures for health care goes for those sixty-five years of age and over. In fact, about one-quarter of total personal health expenditures in the United States from all sources in 1968 was spent for the aged who represent 10 per cent of the population. Per capita, the bill for aged persons was three times the amount for those under sixty-five; $590 versus $195.

Before Medicare, $7 out of every $10 spent for health care of the aged came from private funds. In 1968 only $3 of every $10 came from private funds. In Medicare's first year the program paid for 34 per cent of total medical costs of the aged. By 1968 the proportion was 45 per cent. Other public programs added another 25 per cent, so that together 70 per cent of the health expenditures for the aged is met from public funds.

Comparatively we appear to be doing reasonably well for our older population. The feeling is, however, spreading that there may be an imbalance in our public efforts. There is, for example, a serious relative neglect of children, as I indicated earlier. We don't appear to be doing very well by the remainder of our adult population either.

The United States ranks pretty far down on the list of nations in all comparative health statistics. Most often cited is the fact that we are fifteenth in the list of modern nations in infant mortality (meaning that fourteen nations have lower rates). I am particularly impressed that males in the most productive stage of life, at age forty, have only half as much chance of living to age fifty in the United States as in Sweden, although we spend a much larger share of our GNP on health care than does Sweden. We are eighteenth among nations in life expectancy for males, at birth.

In speaking of the imbalance, I am not suggesting reduction in help for the aged. I would, however, suggest that from now on efforts for the most effective health care assistance for the aged must take serious account of the population as a whole, for many reasons of which I will mention only two. (1) The aged use the same health delivery system as the rest of us. Unless the quality and price problems of the system as a whole are attended to, pouring additional monies into health care for the aged may not really do much effective good for that sector of the population. (2) If increased costs and an inadequate delivery system make access to satisfactory health care a larger burden on the general population, we may see a backlash reaction of resentment against the imbalance. This would be unfortunate for everybody.

Thus, I believe that those who are primarily professionally concerned with improving the lives of our senior citizens would be well advised to consider whether the time has not arrived when they must cease to think in fragmented terms in relation to health care for the aged and to recognize that the solution to their problems is tightly tied to a solution for everybody else.

In short, if we all now think and act as a single community and recognize the inescapable interdependence of persons, as well as health care effectiveness, we are likely to do better for every segment of our population. There is much to be done, and each of us can help.

The Economic Impact of Chronic Diseases

by DOROTHY P. RICE

I AM HAPPY to have this opportunity to partici-
pate in the University of Florida's Annual Southern Conference on
Gerontology to discuss the cost of chronic illness and its impact on
the economy. In this paper, I will present data on the annual expenditures for medical care of chronic disorders affecting almost
half of our total population and more than seven out of ten persons age forty-five years and over. In addition to discussing their
annual direct expenditures for medical care, I will cover the indirect costs or the value of the losses in output to the economy resulting from chronic illnesses.

EXTENT OF CHRONIC ILLNESSES

Medical advances in the prevention and control of formerly
fatally infectious diseases such as pneumonia, typhoid fever, and
tuberculosis have made it possible for an increasing number of
Americans to reach an age at which they become more vulnerable
to arthritis, rheumatism, heart disease, cancer, and other chronic
illnesses. As a result, chronic diseases causing limited or total disability now constitute a major health problem.

An estimated 96 million persons, or 49.9 per cent of the civilian

27

noninstitutionalized population, reported one or more chronic conditions for the twelve-month period ending June, 1967 (Table 1).[1] Although aged people as a group are more prone to suffer chronic illness than those in younger age groups, these illnesses are not limited to the aged population. About 29 per cent of persons under age twenty-five report one or more chronic conditions, compared with 59 per cent of those age twenty-five to forty-four years, 72 per cent in the age group forty-five to sixty-four years, and 86 per cent age sixty-five years and over.

Not all chronic conditions are necessarily disabling although such conditions often require medical care. Of the 85.7 million persons with one or more chronic conditions in July 1963–June 1965, 22.6 million, or more than one-fourth, report some degree of activity limitation.[2]

The following statistics serve to underscore the prevalence and incidence of specific chronic conditions:

—A total of 14.6 million adults have definite heart disease and another 13 million have suspected heart disease.[3]

—About 13 million Americans suffer from some form of arthritis, the nation's number one crippler.[4]

—There are 2.4 million known diabetics in this country.[5]

—Approximately 1.3 million persons have some visual impairment which results in a limitation of activity.[6]

—Approximately 600,000 new cancer cases were diagnosed for

1. U.S. Department of Health, Education, and Welfare, National Center for Health Statistics, *Current Estimates From the Health Interview Survey, United States, July 1966–June 1967*, Public Health Service Publication No. 1000, Series 10, No. 43, January, 1968.

2. U.S. Department of Health, Education, and Welfare, National Center for Health Statistics, *Chronic Conditions Causing Activity Limitation, United States, July 1963–June 1965*, Public Health Service Publication No. 1000, Series 10, No. 51, February, 1969.

3. U.S. Department of Health, Education, and Welfare, National Center for Health Statistics, *Heart Disease in Adults*, Public Health Service Publication No. 1000, Series 11, No. 6, September, 1964.

4. U.S. Department of Health, Education, and Welfare, Public Health Service, *Arthritis: Billion Dollar Crippler*, No. 1444-A, April, 1966.

5. U.S. Department of Health, Education, and Welfare, National Center for Health Statistics, *Characteristics of Persons with Diabetes, United States, July 1964–June 1965*, Public Health Service Publication No. 1000, Series 10, No. 40, October, 1967.

6. *Chronic Conditions Causing Activity Limitation.*

TABLE 1

PERSONS WITH ONE OR MORE CHRONIC CONDITIONS
JULY, 1964–JUNE, 1965

Sex and Age	Total Population (000's)	Persons With One or More Chronic Conditions Number (000's)	Percentage of Population
Both sexes			
All ages	192,359	96,036	49.9
Under 17	67,001	15,564	23.2
17–24	23,074	10,286	44.6
25–44	45,149	26,713	59.2
45–64	39,270	28,112	71.6
65 and over	17,865	15,361	86.0
Male			
All ages	92,803	45,236	48.7
Under 17	34,080	8,379	24.6
17–24	10,641	4,720	44.4
25–44	21,515	12,276	57.1
45–64	18,806	13,248	70.4
65 and over	7,761	6,613	85.2
Female			
All ages	99,557	50,799	51.0
Under 17	32,921	7,185	21.8
17–24	12,433	5,566	44.8
25–44	23,634	14,437	61.1
45–64	20,465	14,863	72.6
65 and over	10,104	8,748	86.6

Source: U.S. Department of Health, Education, and Welfare, Public Health Service. *Current Estimates From the Health Interview Survey, United States, July 1966–June, 1967*. Public Health Service Publication No. 1000, Series 10, No. 43.

the first time in 1969, and 900,000 cases were under medical care for the disease.[7]

—An estimated 17 million adults in the United States have hypertension and 10.5 million adults have hypertensive heart disease.[8]

7. American Cancer Society, *Cancer Facts and Figures*, 1969.
8. U.S. Department of Health, Education, and Welfare, National Center for Health Statistics, *Hypertension and Hypertensive Heart Disease*, Public Health Service Publication No. 1000, Series 11, No. 13, May, 1966.

Health Care Services for the Aged

ANNUAL DIRECT COSTS

What do these numbers mean in terms of dollars and cents? What part of our national expenditures for health and medical care is for care and treatment of these and other chronic illnesses? What are the indirect costs associated with chronic illnesses?[9]

Total expenditures for health and medical care amounted to $34.3 billion in 1963, representing 5.8 per cent of GNP (Table 2).[10] Expenditures for medical care have increased significantly since 1963—from $34.3 billion to $57.1 billion in 1968.[11] Nevertheless, the distribution of these expenditures among the various diagnostic groups has probably remained relatively stable. This paper summarizes the data for 1963, the base year for a detailed study of the cost of illness in the United States.[12]

The allocation of funds by disease is limited in this discussion to the following expenditure categories: hospital and nursing home care, and services of physicians, dentists, and other health professionals. In 1963, these expenditures amounted to $22.5 billion, or approximately two-thirds of the total outlay for health and medical care. The remaining one-third includes a variety of personal and nonpersonal expenditures, including drugs, eyeglasses and appliances, medical research, construction, governmental public health activities, and other miscellaneous expenditures. This latter group of services, not allocated according to disease, includes expenditures for a variety of conditions and illnesses not readily identifiable.

The estimated distribution of 1963 expenditures for specified health services is presented for the eighteen major diagnostic

9. U.S. Senate, Special Committee on Aging, *A Report of the Subcommittee on Health of the Elderly*, "Detection and Prevention of Chronic Disease Utilizing Multiphasic Health Screening Techniques," 89th Cong., 2d sess., U.S. Government Printing Office, December 30, 1966.

10. U.S. Department of Health, Education, and Welfare, Social Security Administration, *Research and Statistics Note No. 10*, 1965, "National Expenditures for Health Care Purposes by Object of Expenditures and Source of Funds, 1960–1963."

11. Dorothy P. Rice and Barbara S. Cooper, "National Health Expenditures, 1929–1969," *Social Security Bulletin*, Vol. 33, No. 1, January, 1970.

12. For details of the study, see Dorothy P. Rice, *Estimating the Cost of Illness*, U.S. Department of Health, Education, and Welfare, Public Health Service Publication No. 947–6, Health Economics Series No. 6, May, 1966.

groups, categorized according to the International Classification of Diseases, Adopted (ICDA). These major diagnostic groups were further classified into chronic and acute categories. Since most of the major diagnostic groups include a mixture of both types of illnesses, the allocation was made on the basis of each group's pre-

TABLE 2

NATIONAL HEALTH EXPENDITURES, 1963

OBJECT OF EXPENDITURE	AMOUNT (MILLIONS)	PERCENTAGE DISTRIBUTION
TOTAL	$34,263	100.0
Personal services and supplies	$29,394	85.5
Hospital care	11,579	33.8
Nursing home care	825	2.4
Physicians' services	6,867	20.0
Dentists' services	2,369	6.9
Other professional services	890	2.6
Drug and drug sundries	4,335	12.7
Eyeglasses and appliances	1,439	4.2
School health services	150	.4
Industrial inplant health services	298	.9
Medical activities in Federal units other than hospitals	642	1.9
Nonpersonal services	4,869	14.2
Medical research	1,195	3.5
Construction	1,566	4.6
Government public health activities[a]	786	2.3
Voluntary health agencies	251	.7
Net cost of insurance	1,071	3.1

Source: U.S. Department of Health, Education, and Welfare, Social Security Administration, *Research and Statistics Note No. 10-1965.* "National Expenditures for Health Care Purposes by Object of Expenditures and Source of Funds, 1960–1963."

a. May include some expenditures for personal services, such as immunization programs.

dominant characteristics. For example, although diseases of the respiratory system include chronic bronchitis, this category is classified as acute because most of the other specific illnesses are, in fact, of the acute type. Likewise, diseases of the digestive system are classified as acute even though they include ulcer and hernia

31

and several other chronic conditions. The Appendix includes a listing of the major diagnostic categories classified according to acute and chronic illnesses and selected subclassifications within each major diagnostic group.

On the basis of this admittedly rough classification system, expenditures for medical care and treatment of chronic conditions amounted to the staggering sum of more than $12 billion in 1963, or 53 per cent of the total personal health care expenditures distributed among the various diseases (Table 3). Not included here are other direct costs such as amounts spent for drugs and for research in chronic diseases, which would make the total even greater.

There are striking differences among the several expenditure categories in terms of the diagnostic distributions. Expenditures for chronic illnesses account for 62 per cent of the hospital care, but only 51 per cent of physicians' services. As expected, a major portion of the expenditures for nursing homes, 82 per cent, is for care of chronic conditions. Only a small proportion, 21 per cent, of payments for the services of other professional personnel represents expenditures for chronic illnesses. Included in this category are dental services which are classified under acute conditions.

ANNUAL INDIRECT COSTS

These statistics point up the fact that a substantial portion of the nation's annual health expenditures is spent for hospital and medical care of persons with chronic illnesses. However, direct expenditures do not measure the full economic costs imposed upon the nation by illness, disability, and premature death since they do not include the loss of output to the economy. These losses, labeled indirect costs, are perhaps even more arresting.

Chronic illnesses causing limitation of activity, institutionalization, and death result in losses of output to the economy. The vast majority of the 1.5 million persons in institutions are there because of some chronic disability. More than 70 per cent of deaths are now due to three chronic illnesses—heart disease, cancer, and stroke. A total of 224 million days was lost from work in 1963 due to chronic conditions.

32

In addition to persons in the labor force who occasionally do not work because of illness and disability, there is a considerable number of individuals not in institutions who are unable to work. It is true that not all of them would have worked or been productive if illness had not interfered. Some are too old or too young for gainful employment. Others are unwilling to work and some are unable to find a job. Nevertheless, a reasonable estimate of the value of their losses in output can be made by assuming that if it were not for these illnesses, these stricken persons would have had the same employment experience as persons in the same age and sex group under conditions of full employment. If full employment is not assumed, losses due to death and disability cannot be isolated from losses due to unemployment. The calculation of the annual loss in output is performed by applying prevailing average earnings to the productive time lost by age and sex group for each major cause of death and major type of illness.

An important group usually overlooked in estimating illness costs is the female keeping house. In 1963, a total 323,000 women were reported unable to keep house because of illness. A value has been imputed to housewives' services equal to the average yearly earnings of a domestic worker, or $2,670 in 1963. This imputed value is clearly on the low side because it makes no allowance for the housewife's longer work week and does not take into account the size of the household cared for.

A total of 6.2 million man-years was lost in 1963 due to death and illness. As previously indicated, not all of these years would have been productive. Of this total, three-fourths (4.6 million man-years) represent productive years lost, valued at $23.8 billion.

ANNUAL INDIRECT COSTS OF CHRONIC ILLNESSES

Using the rough classification system outlined above, the values of losses in output were also classified according to chronic and acute conditions. More than three-fifths of the annual indirect costs, valued at $15.1 billion, are associated with chronic conditions (Table 4). The distribution of these indirect costs according to population group reveals some significant differences between acute and chronic conditions.

TABLE 3

NATIONAL HEALTH EXPENDITURES—SELECTED CATEGORIES, 1963

Diagnosis	Total	Hospital Care	Nursing Home Care	Professional Services	
				Physicians	Other[b]
Total (in millions)	$22,530.0	$11,579.0	$825.0	$6,867.0	$3,259.0
			Percentage distribution		
Total	100.0	100.0	100.0	100.0	100.0
Chronic conditions, total	53.4	62.0	81.8	51.1	21.0
Tuberculosis	1.1	2.0		2.2	.1
Neoplasms	5.7	8.7	3.3	3.0	1.2
Allergic, endocrine, metabolic and nutritional diseases	4.0	2.9	3.4	7.5	.6
Diseases of blood and blood-forming organs	.7	.5		1.4	.2
Mental, psychoneurotic and personality disorders	10.7	17.8	3.6	4.1	.9
Diseases of nervous system and sense organs	6.3	5.9	21.6	7.4	1.4
Diseases of circulatory system	10.1	11.0	25.1	10.4	2.2
Diseases of genitourinary system	5.4	6.4	1.5	6.3	.8
Diseases of bones and organs of movement	6.3	4.3	6.3	6.6	13.0
Congenital malformations	.5	.8		.3	.1
Symptoms, senility, and ill-defined conditions	2.8	1.7	17.0	4.0	.3
Acute conditions, total	46.6	38.0	18.2	48.9	79.0
Infective and parasitic diseases	1.2	.9		2.1	.2
Diseases of the respiratory system	7.0	6.5		11.7	.8

Diseases of the digestive system	18.5	11.5	1.1	5.8	74.1[c]
Maternity	6.2	7.9		6.2	1.4
Diseases of skin and cellular tissue	1.1	1.3		1.4	.2
Certain diseases of early infancy	.1	.2		.1	a
Injuries	7.6	8.6	8.8	8.8	.9
Miscellaneous	5.0	1.1	8.3	12.8	1.3

Source: Dorothy P. Rice, *Estimating the Cost of Illness*, Department of Health, Education, and Welfare, Public Health Service Publication No. 947–6. Health Economics Series No. 6, May, 1966.

a. Less than .05 per cent.

b. Includes nursing care and services of dentists, podiatrists, physical therapists, clinical psychologists, chiropractors, naturopaths, and Christian Science practitioners.

c. Includes dental care.

TABLE 4
ANNUAL MORTALITY AND MORBIDITY LOSSES—INDIRECT COSTS BY POPULATION GROUPS, 1963

DIAGNOSIS	TOTAL	MORTALITY	MORBIDITY	
			INSTITU-TIONAL	NON-INSTITU-TIONAL
Total (in millions)	$23,773.1	$2,731.0	$5,104.3	$15,937.9
		PERCENTAGE DISTRIBUTION		
Total	100.0	100.0	100.0	100.0
Chronic conditions, total	63.7	80.8	96.1	50.4
Tuberculosis	1.7	.7	2.8	1.5
Neoplasms	5.6	17.7	1.1	5.0
Allergic, endocrine, metabolic and nutritional diseases	2.6	2.5	1.1	3.0
Diseases of blood and blood-forming organs	.2	.3	.1	.2
Mental, psychoneurotic and personality disorders	19.5	.4	71.3	6.2
Diseases of nervous system and sense organs	7.7	11.0	6.0	7.6
Diseases of circulatory system	17.4	44.9	6.4	16.3
Diseases of genitourinary system	2.3	1.8	.3	3.0
Diseases of bones and organs of movement	5.2	.2	1.6	7.2
Congenital malformations	.2	.2		.3
Symptoms, senility, and ill-defined conditions	1.4	1.2	5.3	.1
Acute conditions, total	36.3	19.2	3.9	49.6
Infective and parasitic diseases	2.0	.5	a	3.0
Diseases of the respiratory system	13.9	5.1	.2	19.8

Diseases of the digestive system	5.7	4.5	.4	7.5
Maternity	.1	.1		.2
Diseases of skin and cellular tissue	.6	.1	a	.8
Certain diseases of early infancy				
Injuries	8.6	8.9	2.1	10.7
Miscellaneous	5.4		1.3	7.6

Source: Same as for Table 3.
a. Less than .05 per cent.

As expected, losses for persons who died from all chronic conditions such as cancer, diseases of the circulatory system, and diseases of the nervous system, represent more than four-fifths of the mortality dollar losses. Because institutionalized persons are largely afflicted with chronic illnesses, their losses in output represent almost all of the institutional losses—96 per cent of the total. For the noninstitutionalized population, including the currently employed, those unable to work, and women keeping house, chronic diseases account for more than half of the total losses in output— $8 billion out of $15.9 billion. Diseases of the circulatory system, the nervous system and sense organs, and diseases of the bones and organs of movement (including arthritis) represent a significantly high proportion of the chronic disease losses for the noninstitutionalized population.

AGE DISTRIBUTION

Although the incidence and severity of chronic diseases increases with age, these chronic conditions and the resulting losses in output are by no means limited to the aged. The distribution by age shows that dollar losses are highest for those age forty-five to sixty-four, accounting for $6.9 billion, or 45 per cent of the $15.1 billion annual indirect costs of chronic illnesses (Table 5). Productivity losses for the sixty-five and over age group represent a considerably smaller proportion of the total, 26 per cent, reflecting the relatively lower productivity of this age group.

ANNUAL ECONOMIC COST

The total annual economic cost of all illnesses—the sum of the direct expenditures for medical care and the indirect costs of illness, disability, and death—was estimated at $58 billion in 1963 and was comprised of the following: (1) $34.3 billion spent for medical care, services, and supplies. Of this total, $22.5 billion was distributed among the major diagnostic groups. (2) $23.8 billion lost to the economy in 1963 due to premature death, illness, and disability for all diseases. Of the $46.3 billion total economic cost distributed among the major diagnostic groups, $27.2 billion, or almost three-fifths, represents the annual costs of chronic illnesses (Table 6).

38

TABLE 5

ANNUAL MORTALITY AND MORBIDITY LOSSES—INDIRECT COSTS BY AGE GROUPS, 1963

DIAGNOSIS	ALL AGES	UNDER 25	25–44	45–64	65 AND OVER
Total (in millions)	$23,773.1	$1,113.4	$7,143.1	$10,733.5	$4,783.2
		PERCENTAGE DISTRIBUTION			
Total	100.0	100.0	100.0	100.0	100.0
Chronic conditions, total	63.7	45.3	53.8	64.1	81.8
Tuberculosis	1.7	2.1	2.2	1.7	.9
Neoplasms	5.6	3.6	3.7	6.3	7.3
Allergic, endocrine, metabolic and nutritional diseases	2.6	1.8	2.0	2.9	2.7
Diseases of blood and blood-forming organs	.2	.2	.2	.1	.3
Mental, psychoneurotic and personality disorders	19.5	21.9	25.5	17.7	14.0
Diseases of nervous system and sense organs	7.7	6.2	4.8	6.8	14.2
Diseases of circulatory system	17.4	3.7	7.6	19.2	31.3
Diseases of genitourinary system	2.3	2.1	2.7	2.3	1.8
Diseases of bones and organs of movement	5.2	2.9	4.5	6.0	5.0
Congenital malformations	.2	.4	.3	.2	.1
Symptoms, senility, and ill-defined conditions	1.4	.3	.4	.8	4.2
Acute conditions, total	36.3	54.7	46.2	35.9	18.2
Infective and parasitic diseases	2.0	5.1	2.9	1.9	.4
Diseases of the respiratory system	13.9	19.3	17.4	14.3	6.5
Diseases of the digestive system	5.7	6.2	6.3	6.2	3.3
Maternity	.1	1.4	.3	a	
Diseases of skin and cellular tissue	.6	1.5	.5	.6	.3
Certain diseases of early infancy					
Injuries	8.6	15.0	12.6	7.2	4.5
Miscellaneous	5.3	6.2	6.3	5.6	3.2

Source: Same as for Table 3.
a. Less than .05 per cent.

39

Health Care Services for the Aged

TABLE 6

ANNUAL ECONOMIC COST—ESTIMATED DIRECT EXPENDITURES
AND INDIRECT COSTS OF MORBIDITY AND
MORTALITY, 1963

Diagnosis	Total	Direct Expenditures	Indirect Costs
Total	$46,303.1	$22,530.0	$23,773.1
	Percentage distribution		
Total	100.0	100.0	100.0
Chronic conditions, total	58.7	53.4	63.7
Tuberculosis	1.4	1.1	1.7
Neoplasms	5.6	5.7	5.6
Allergic, endocrine, metabolic and nutritional diseases	3.3	4.0	2.6
Diseases of blood and blood-forming organs	.4	.7	.2
Mental, psychoneurotic and personality disorders	15.2	10.7	19.5
Diseases of nervous system and sense organs	7.0	6.3	7.7
Diseases of circulatory system	13.8	10.1	17.4
Diseases of genitourinary system	3.8	5.4	2.3
Diseases of bones and organs of movement	5.7	6.3	5.2
Congenital malformations	.3	.5	.2
Symptoms, senility, and ill-defined conditions	2.0	2.8	1.4
Acute conditions, total	41.3	46.6	36.3
Infective and parasitic diseases	1.6	1.2	2.0
Diseases of the respiratory system	10.6	7.0	13.9
Diseases of the digestive system	11.9	18.5	5.7
Maternity	3.1	6.2	.1
Diseases of skin and cellular tissue	.8	1.1	.6
Certain diseases of early infancy	.1	.1	
Injuries	8.1	7.6	8.6
Miscellaneous	5.1	5.0	5.3

Source: Same as for Table 3.

40

ECONOMIC COST OF MORTALITY

Although the annual direct and indirect costs of illnesses are high from the economist's point of view, single-year cost estimates represent only part of the estimated losses in output resulting from illness, disability, and death. If an individual who died this year had not succumbed, he would have continued to be productive for a number of years. If he is ill and disabled this year and his disability continues into future years, his future productivity will be affected. It is the present value of these future losses that constitutes the appropriate measure of the costs of a disease. For mortality, the estimated cost or value to society of deaths in a particular year is the product of the number of deaths in that year and the expected value of these individuals' future earnings after sex and age have been taken into account. This method of derivation must consider life expectancy for different age and sex groups, the changing pattern of earnings at successive ages, varying labor force participation rates, imputed value of housewives' services, and the appropriate discount rate to convert a stream of costs or benefits into its present worth.[13]

Applying these expected lifetime earnings by age and sex, as shown in Table 7, to the 1.8 million deaths in 1963 results in a loss of nearly $50 billion to the economy, at a 4 per cent discount rate. These deaths represent a loss of 32.5 million man-years. For the 1.4 million persons who died from chronic diseases, an estimated total of almost 20 million man-years was lost, valued at $32.8 billion (Table 8). Thus, almost two-thirds of the estimated lifetime earnings lost from all deaths in 1963 are attributed to chronic disease deaths.

AGE DISTRIBUTION

Of the 1.8 million deaths, the highest proportion was naturally among the aged, with those age sixty-five years and over representing three-fifths of the total. The forty-five to sixty-four age group is also strongly represented among the deaths, comprising

13. Dorothy P. Rice, "The Economic Value of Human Life," *The American Journal of Public Health* 57 (November 1967): 1954–66.

41

nearly one-fourth of the total. In terms of lost lifetime earnings, however, the latter age group accounted for two-fifths and the sixty-five and over age group accounted for only one-fifth of the total amount. The much higher earnings losses for those who died in the forty-five to sixty-four age group are due to their considerably higher expected earnings.

The age distribution of losses for those who died from chronic diseases shows a similar pattern. Of the 1.4 million who died due to these conditions, one-fourth were age forty-five to sixty-four and 67 per cent were age sixty-five and over. The lifetime earnings

TABLE 7

PRESENT VALUE OF LIFETIME EARNINGS[a]

Age	Males	Females
Under 1	$59,063	$34,622
1–4	64,989	37,938
5–9	79,333	46,289
10–14	96,736	56,422
15–19	114,613	64,936
20–24	126,688	67,960
25–29	128,698	66,826
30–34	122,904	64,389
35–39	111,956	60,998
40–44	97,301	56,603
45–49	80,325	50,896
50–54	63,027	44,371
55–59	45,948	37,467
60–64	28,387	30,164
65–69	15,043	23,579
70–74	9,264	18,118
75–79	5,344	12,888
80–84	2,935	6,916
85 and over	210	1,123

Source: Same as for Table 3.

a. Represents present value of expected lifetime earnings for projected fatalities in each year, calculated for each five-year age and sex group on the basis of 1963 life tables, 1963 labor force participation rates adjusted for full employment (an average 4 per cent unemployment rate), 1963 mean earnings, imputed value of housewives' services, 1963 housekeeping rates, and an annual net effective discount rate of 4 per cent.

TABLE 8

TOTAL MORTALITY LOSSES BY DEATHS, YEARS LOST, AND
LIFETIME EARNINGS, 1963

Diagnosis	Number of Deaths	Total Years Lost (in thousands)	Lifetime Earnings (millions)
Total	1,812,921	32,533.0	$49,928.1
	Percentage distribution		
Total	100.0	100.0	100.0
Chronic conditions, total	78.8	61.3	65.8
Tuberculosis	.5	.5	.7
Neoplasms	16.0	14.6	16.9
Allergic, endocrine, metabolic and nutritional diseases	2.4	2.1	2.4
Diseases of blood and blood-forming organs	.3	.4	.4
Mental, psychoneurotic and personality disorders	.3	.4	.5
Diseases of nervous system and sense organs	11.9	7.9	7.7
Diseases of circulatory system	43.1	27.9	31.6
Diseases of genitourinary system	1.7	1.5	1.7
Diseases of bones and organs of movement	.2	.2	.3
Congenital malformations	1.1	4.1	2.2
Symptoms, senility and ill-defined conditions	1.2	1.6	1.5
Acute conditions, total	21.2	38.7	34.2
Infective and parasitic diseases	.6	1.0	.9
Diseases of the respiratory system	5.8	6.7	5.3
Diseases of the digestive system	4.0	4.4	4.9
Maternity	.1	.2	.2
Diseases of skin and cellular tissue	.1	.1	.1
Certain diseases of early infancy	3.5	13.5	6.2
Injuries	7.2	12.8	16.6

Source: Same as for Table 3.

TABLE 9

TOTAL MORTALITY LOSSES—VALUE OF LIFETIME EARNINGS BY AGE, 1963

Diagnosis	All Ages	Under 25	25–44	45–64	65 and Over
Total (in millions)	$49,928.1	$10,195.6	$9,753.8	$19,870.3	$10,108.4
			Percentage distribution		
Total	100.0	100.0	100.0	100.0	100.0
Chronic conditions, total	65.8	25.0	55.1	80.5	88.2
Tuberculosis	.7	.2	1.1	.9	.4
Neoplasms	16.9	5.5	16.0	23.0	17.4
Allergic, endocrine, metabolic and nutritional diseases	2.4	.9	2.5	2.6	3.1
Diseases of blood and blood-forming organs	.4	.6	.4	.2	.3
Mental, psychoneurotic and personality disorders	.5	.4	1.1	.5	.1
Diseases of nervous system and sense organs	7.7	3.1	5.8	7.7	14.2
Diseases of circulatory system	31.6	1.8	22.6	41.9	49.8
Diseases of genitourinary system	1.7	1.0	2.5	1.7	1.6
Diseases of bones and organs of movement	.3	.4	.2	.2	.2
Congenital malformations	2.2	9.2	.9	.3	.1
Symptoms, senility and ill-defined conditions	1.5	2.0	1.9	1.3	.9
Acute conditions, total	34.2	75.0	44.9	19.5	11.8
Infective and parasitic diseases	.9	1.9	.9	.6	.4
Diseases of the respiratory system	5.3	8.7	3.8	4.5	5.1
Diseases of the digestive system	4.9	3.2	6.3	5.9	3.4
Maternity	.2	.3	.7	•	
Diseases of skin and cellular tissue	.1	.1	.2	.1	.1
Certain diseases of early infancy	6.2	30.1			
Injuries	16.6	30.7	33.1	8.3	2.8

a. Less than .05 per cent.
Source: Same as Table 3.

TABLE 10

TOTAL ECONOMIC COST, 1963 (*Discounted at 4 per cent*)

DIAGNOSIS	TOTAL	DIRECT EXPENDITURES	MORBIDITY	TOTAL MORTALITY
Total (in millions)	$93,500.3	$22,530.0	$21,042.2	$49,928.1
		PERCENTAGE DISTRIBUTION		
Total	100.0	100.0	100.0	100.0
Chronic conditions, total	61.8	53.4	61.5	65.8
Tuberculosis	1.0	1.1	1.8	.7
Neoplasms	11.3	5.7	4.0	16.9
Allergic, endocrine, metabolic and nutritional diseases	2.8	4.0	2.6	2.4
Diseases of blood and blood forming organs	.4	.7	.2	.4
Mental, psychoneurotic and personality disorders	7.8	10.7	22.0	.5
Diseases of nervous system and sense organs	7.3	6.3	7.2	7.7
Diseases of circulatory systems	22.4	10.1	13.9	31.6
Diseases of genitourinary system	2.7	5.4	2.4	1.7
Diseases of bones and organs of movement	3.0	6.3	5.8	.3
Congenital malformations	1.3	.5	.2	2.2
Symptoms, senility and ill-defined conditions	1.8	2.8	1.4	1.5
Acute conditions, total	38.2	46.6	38.5	34.2
Infective and parasitic diseases	1.2	1.2	2.2	.9
Diseases of the respiratory system	7.9	7.0	15.0	5.3
Diseases of the digestive system	8.4	18.5	5.8	4.9
Maternity	1.6	6.2	.2	.2
Diseases of skin and cellular tissue	.5	1.1	.6	.1
Certain diseases of early infancy	3.3	.1		6.2
Injuries	12.6	7.6	8.6	16.6
Miscellaneous	2.5	5.0	6.1	

Source: Same as for Table 3.

losses once again show a reverse relationship: losses are considerably higher for the former group.

The distribution of lifetime earnings losses within each age group shows that the proportion for chronic diseases increases sharply with advancing age (Table 9).

TOTAL COSTS

Summing up the annual direct expenditures for illnesses, annual morbidity costs, and lifetime earnings losses due to death in 1963, the total economic cost amounts to $93.5 billion, at a 4 per cent discount rate (Table 10). The distribution according to chronic and acute conditions shows that losses resulting from the former are considerably greater than the latter. The economic toll associated with illness, disability, and death in 1963 due to chronic diseases amounts to $57.8 billion, a rather staggering amount by any definition.

APPENDIX

LISTING OF MAJOR DIAGNOSTIC CATEGORIES AND
SELECTED SUBCLASSIFICATIONS

CHRONIC CONDITIONS

Tuberculosis
Neoplasms
Allergic, endocrine, metabolic, and nutritional diseases
    Allergic disorders
    Diseases of thyroid gland
    Diabetes mellitus
    Diseases of other endocrine glands
    Avitaminoses and other metabolic diseases
Diseases of blood and blood-forming organs
    Anemia
    Hemophilia
    Diseases of spleen
Mental, psychoneurotic, and personality disorders
Diseases of the nervous system and sense organs
    Vascular lesions affecting central nervous system (stroke)
    Inflammatory and other diseases of central nervous system
    Diseases of nerves and peripheral ganglia

Inflammatory and other diseases of eye
Diseases of ear and mastoid process
Diseases of the circulatory system
    Rheumatic fever and rheumatic heart disease
    Arteriosclerotic and other diseases of the heart
    Hypertension
    Diseases of arteries
    Diseases of veins and other diseases of circulatory system
Diseases of the genitourinary system
    Nephritis and nephrosis
    Other diseases of urinary system
    Diseases of male genital organs
    Diseases of female genital organs
Diseases of bones and organs of movement
    Arthritis and rheumatism
    Osteomyelitis and other diseases of bone and joint
    Other diseases of musculoskeletal system
Congenital malformations
    Monstrosity
    Congenital malformations of circulatory system
    Cleft palate and harelip
Symptoms, senility, and ill-defined conditions
    Symptoms referable to systems or organs
    Senility and ill-defined conditions

ACUTE CONDITIONS

Infective and parasitic diseases
    Venereal diseases
    Diseases attributable to viruses
    Typhus and other rickettsial diseases
    Malaria
Diseases of the respiratory system
    Acute upper respiratory infections
    Influenza
    Pneumonia
    Bronchitis, acute and chronic
    Other diseases of respiratory system
Diseases of the digestive system
    Diseases of buccal cavity and esophagus (dental conditions)
    Diseases of stomach and duodenum
    Appendicitis
    Hernia of abdominal cavity
    Diseases of liver, gallbladder and pancreas
Pregnancy, childbirth, puerperium (maternity)
Diseases of skin and cellular tissue
Certain diseases of early infancy
    Birth injuries, asphyxia, and infections of newborn
    Other diseases peculiar to early infancy
Injuries and adverse effects of chemical and other external causes

The Hospital of the Seventies

by ANNE R. SOMERS

CRYSTAL-GAZING, as everyone knows, is a hazard-ous occupation. Cassandra was all-too-correct in her prediction of ill-fortune for the ancient Greeks, but she paid for her foresight with her life and the legend that bears her name still gives pause to would-be readers of political and economic tea leaves.

Nevertheless, the need for information as to probable future developments, as a basis for business and institutional planning, is now so great and the financial and political stakes are so high that a whole new profession of "futurists" has emerged. Armed with computers, regression equations, and other statistical and elec-tronic aides, they boldly set out to project the world as they see it—five, ten, even twenty-five years ahead.

The projections are often wrong. But still it's fun, it's good men-tal exercise, and I am sure that, on balance, it does more good than harm. For one thing, it gets us into the habit of looking forward rather than backward and that in itself is a real gain.

So, here, for your consideration is a model of the community hospital as I see it evolving over the past two decades and through the decade of the seventies—a purely theoretical model but one which I hope may help to clarify some of the many seemingly con-tradictory trends.

48

THE MODEL

The hospital of the mid-seventies will be the central coordinating force—the organizational hub—of the entire system of community health services. When I say hospital I mean all the elements in that complex institution—the trustees, the medical staff, the administration, the nursing service, etc. By community health services I mean all the professionally controlled services provided to substantial numbers of people in what may be called the mainstream of care and regardless of whether they are financed primarily on a public or private basis.

This does *not* mean that all such services will be physically provided within the hospital. On the contrary, the community health system of the future will not only require fewer hospital beds, per capita, than at present but will stress physical decentralization for all services except those that actually require sophisticated technological equipment and highly specialized personnel. There will be increasing emphasis on neighborhood health centers—these, I believe, will be located in affluent as well as underprivileged neighborhoods—on private group practice clinics, on first-aid stations in isolated localities, on good long-term care facilities, home health services, etc.

It does mean that the hospital—as the broadest based source of authority, in terms of professional, technological, and financial resources, the site where professional needs and values and community needs and values meet and can be reconciled—will be assigned responsibility for assuring the essential functional and organizational relationships and the necessary qualitative and quantitative controls to make the whole complex system of community health services work on a predominantly voluntary basis.

What do these words mean in practice? Obviously, in a country of this size and wide regional and cultural variations, they will mean different things in different places. But, at the risk of great over-simplification, here are two illustrations. I am assuming throughout this discussion an evolutionary development, with all this implies in terms of some continuing irrationalities, rather than a drastic revolutionary overhauling of our present nonsystem—an overhauling that might well lose more than it would gain.

49

MERCY COMMUNITY HOSPITAL

Mercy is a typical community hospital of the mid-seventies, one of six serving a highly urbanized city of about 500,000, which I will call Urbanton. Urbanton does not really need six hospitals. Four would be quite adequate and more in line with the national trend to fewer, larger institutions. However, until 1971, there were seven separate hospitals in this community and the reduction to six, by merger of two, represents progress.

Mercy has about 350 beds, a first-class surgical service, an intensive-care unit, a coronary care unit, and a renal dialysis unit. The department of ambulatory services includes most of the usual specialty clinics, a physical rehabilitation service, a geriatric clinic emphasizing psychiatric services, a well-developed social service, a small but excellent emergency service, and a first-class primary care unit. There are no inpatient pediatric or maternity services.

In addition to these central facilities, Mercy operates a 200-bed extended care facility, just a few blocks away, two neighborhood health centers—one and three miles from the hospital respectively—and an extensive home health service. It has referral agreements with two additional ECF's, several nursing homes, and a community mental health center.

Most of its nonprofessional services—laundry, food services, housekeeping, business operations—and even some of the professional—most of the routine laboratory work for example—are provided through a multi-hospital corporation contracting with the six hospitals.

The medical staff consists of approximately 150 physicians, about 50 of whom are full-time. These include the medical director, director of medical education, director of community medicine, chiefs of all the major services, the radiology, pathology, anesthesiology, physical medicine, and psychiatry departments in toto, the staffs of the emergency room, primary care unit, and the two satellite neighborhood health centers.

Most of the doctors have their offices in the medical arts building next door to the hospital and owned by it. The largest suite is occupied by the Mercy Medical Group—a separate organization of thirty-five physicians. The rest of the building is occupied by doctors in various degrees of combination, mostly two- or three-man partnerships. Nearly all—except for the obstetricians, and pediatricians—have their primary affiliation with Mercy, although many have joint appointments in other hospitals as well.

Mercy is not a teaching hospital in the sense that it has under-graduate medical students. However, it is affiliated with Metro-politan University Hospital, about fifty miles away. Thanks to this affiliation, it has an organized referral system for the super-special-ties, the benefit of easy consultation with the staff of University Hospital, and close working relations with respect to its residency program. This affiliation, plus the hospital's vastly increased inter-est in community medicine, have enabled it to obtain a majority of United States–trained house staff for the past few years, a situation that never prevailed in the sixties.

Mercy's patient population is still not defined as precisely as some planners would like to see. Nevertheless, a pretty clear de facto service area has gradually emerged, particularly as a result of clearer identification of the community's primary care doctors with a single institution.

Since all the hospitals do not provide all services, however, there is necessarily some crossing of geographical boundaries. This latter policy was hotly debated for several years. There were community leaders as well as doctors who felt that every hospital should have a maternity and pediatric service, a cobalt unit, a dialysis unit, an emergency room, in general the whole gamut of hospital services. But eventually those who favored a policy of partial institutional specialization prevailed. Mercy reluctantly gave up its inpatient pediatric and maternity services in return for recognized pre-eminence in geriatric services and the only dialysis unit in Urbanton. It continues to provide ambulatory pediatric and maternity care, through its department of community health, but patients with serious illnesses requiring hospital admission are referred to the Good Neighbor Hospital, only a few miles away and whose facilities and staff have specialized in these areas. As *quid pro quo*, Mercy's dialysis unit and geriatric clinic serve the entire community.

Today, three years after the somewhat traumatic realignment of programs, both physicians and community appear generally pleased with the results. Better services are being provided at less cost than would otherwise have been the case. In the late sixties, Mercy's obstetrics service was running an occupancy of about one-third, Good Neighbor about 50 per cent. Today, the latter's obstetrics rate averages close to 80 per cent—about as high as a maternity service can be expected to operate effectively.

Costs at Mercy are not low. The all-inclusive cost for an in-patient day at Mercy is now $125. Hospital costs have continued to rise but it is hard to compare them with the experience of the sixties since the crude and meaningless "expense per patient day" measure was abandoned several years ago by the American Hospital Association and the United States Bureau of Labor Statistics now prices many other hospital services in addition to the inpatient room rate, thus providing a more realistic picture of hospital costs.

Fortunately, methods of financing care have also continued to develop so that this high price is virtually never borne by an individual patient at the time of illness. Despite mounting pressure for extending Medicare to the entire population this has still not been done, chiefly because private insurers, doctors, and hospitals are now seriously working together in the effort to develop new techniques of spreading the costs, bringing in government financing at many points, but retaining voluntary initiative in design and operation of the programs.

The more affluent of Mercy's patients continue to rely on traditional types of insurance, especially the combination of basic hospital coverage and major medical. Under these plans, physicians are still paid on a fee-for-service basis. The majority of patients, however, are now covered by a new type of prepayment plan, modelled somewhat after the Kaiser Foundation Health Plan, on the West Coast, and now sold by a number of carriers in other parts of the country. Under this scheme, Mercy Hospital and its medical staff provide subscribers with all necessary medical care for a flat monthly fee. The plan acts as fiscal intermediary for a number of groups, including most of the major union health and welfare funds, a number of the principal employers in the area, Medicare, etc.

So far as medical services are involved, some—for example those in the neighborhood health centers—are provided by salaried doctors, for others the hospital contracts with the Mercy Medical Group. Inpatient maternity and pediatric services and highly specialized services such as open heart or brain surgery are purchased by Mercy on behalf of these patients from other institutions with which it has referral agreements.

The financial arrangements are complicated and more expensive than if provided under a single national Medicare plan. However, they are clearly in line with our traditional preference for pluralistic financing, no matter how complicated, rather than outright government operation. In any case, the institution of a capitation approach to payment for hospital and medical costs and their integration into a single program have helped considerably to make doctors more cost conscious, to force hospitals to hold the line on rising costs more firmly, and generally to restrain the rise in costs to bearable dimensions.

METROPOLITAN UNIVERSITY HOSPITAL

Metropolitan University Hospital is one of the nation's hundred best and largest teaching hospitals, the primary teaching arm of a first-rate medical school. With 800 beds it has virtually every major specialty and superspecialty. It also has a large and active department of community and family medicine which is largely responsible for administering the network of affiliations with community hospitals and other community health facilities and programs.

Like Mercy, it also has an active ambulatory service and several neighborhood health centers. Unlike at Mercy, however, these are operated primarily as research, teaching, and demonstration units. They are relatively small and deliberately focused on the most difficult patient populations within reasonable access. For example, one center is located in a skid row area where drug addiction and alcoholism, combined with multiple socioeconomic problems, present University's Department of Community Medicine and Department of Drug and Alcohol Studies with abundant "teaching material" while providing the inhabitants of this area with as good care as can be found anywhere in the country. Patient care for this grossly atypical population is heavily subsidized by a new Institute of Community Medicine in the National Institute of Health.

The ambulatory center in University Hospital itself seeks to present students and faculty with a typical cross-section of the population. The number it serves, however, is deliberately restricted to a number that can be dealt with at the inevitably slower pace required for academic patient care. The costs are paid in the same way as at Mercy—partly by traditional insurance, partly by capitation plans, but in all cases with an educational subsidy. Thus the carriers and subscribers are not charged the extra cost of academic care. The patient population is largely self-selected and comes from a relatively large area of the Metropolis.

University's residents and interns, as well as graduate students in public health and hospital administration, are rotated among several of the affiliated community hospitals, like Mercy. This is especially true of those who are specializing in community or family medicine. Conversely, residents from the community hospitals come into University at frequent intervals for conferences, grand rounds, and once a year for a two-week residency. The interchange between house staff and faculty in the two types of institutions has been enriching to both and has improved the total quality of patient care available in the entire area.

PRIMARY CARE FACILITIES

To complete the picture, one would have to give similar vignettes illustrating the organization and work of institutions that are smaller and less professionally sophisticated than Mercy Hospital. Depending on the cultural and physical geography of the area and region this might be a small rural hospital, a neighborhood health center in a large urban area, a private group practice clinic, an emergency first-aid station in a sparsely populated region or in a seasonal resort area, whose primary facility might be a helicopter or Piper Cub, a college infirmary, a small industrial hospital in the mining or lumbering fields, or any number of other types of primary care units where emergency services must be provided on a standby basis but where the chief requirement in any serious situation is quick transfer to a fully equipped hospital.

The diversity of such institutions and lack of time preclude doing justice to this echelon of the developing health care system.

It should be clear, however, that the organization, staffing, and financing of such services are a vitally important link in the total picture if all Americans are to be provided with good medical care. The time for wishfully thinking that we can persuade good young doctors to move into such areas on a solo basis is already past. By the mid-seventies, let us hope, all efforts will be concentrated on linking these primary outposts of care to our urban hospital system. Let us also hope that the urban hospitals will rise to the challenge of assuming responsibility for these units by developing mutually beneficial satellite agreements.

PRINCIPAL BARRIERS

The Chinese have a saying to the effect that it is easier to paint a dragon than a horse. Many of you are undoubtedly saying that it is much easier to paint these glowing pictures of nonexistent Mercy and University Hospitals than it would be to work out the immediate problems in your real life institutions. Of course you would be right. No one today can be so naïve as to think anything approaching such a community, regional, and ultimately national system of health services can be achieved without overcoming numerous difficulties and probably without having to live through some pretty rough battles and many temporary setbacks.

Let me try to identify some of the major barriers as I see them.

First, and perhaps most obvious, is the fact that very few hospitals in the United States have geographically defined service boundaries. Indeed, many hospitals, especially in multi-hospital urban areas, do not really know what their service area is, or the size of the population they serve, or other elementary facts essential to rational planning and programming.

Whether we will eventually reach a stage where hospital districts are defined as precisely as school districts, I am not sure. I am not even sure I would want to see it. More important than 100 per cent geographical precision is a sense of commitment to a specific community or a portion of a community. And I do feel sure that, as the costs of hospital care continue to rise, we will move generally in this direction. If hospitals do not get together and make at least some informal service area agreements among themselves it will be forced on them from outside.

Second, the problem of financing is of course formidable and is perhaps the major obstacle cited by most hospital spokesmen for failure to move further in the direction of comprehensive care, especially ambulatory. No one knows what the ultimate solution to this problem will be. The easiest way out—especially in the short run—would be to turn the whole problem over to government through the extension of Medicare to the whole population. This will be, I suspect, a real temptation, not only to the public which doesn't much care how the financing is arranged, provided the direct costs are not too great and they are not related to a means test, but also to the providers and carriers who may find the Medicare route appealingly simple compared to the problems and headaches of pluralistic financing. Nevertheless, I still believe that new and ingenious efforts will be made to keep the financing pluralistic, although it is probable that the federal government may have to legislate universal coverage and find some way of augmenting the funds raised through private health insurance. In my picture of Mercy Hospital in 1975 I have suggested one way that the voluntary sector could be strengthened.

Even more difficult than the problem of financing is the problem of hospital–physician relations. In the words of the Catholic Hospital Association's 1968 policy statement on comprehensive care, "The hospital administration–medical staff interface will be the site of maximum strain during this period of health service development."

This is a problem that I dealt with at some length in a rather widely publicized article that appeared in Part 2 of the *Journal of Medical Education,* January, 1965, the proceedings of one of the Association of American Medical Colleges Teaching Institutes. The article dealt with the conflict between Dr. Jones, a conscientious hospital-based physician, and Dr. Smith, equally conscientious but who practiced largely outside the hospital orbit. I concluded, even then, that time, history, and the progress of medical science and technology were on the side of Dr. Jones. I still believe this and think that developments of the past few years have demonstrated the correctness of this position.

But I also believe that there will be, at least for the foreseeable future, a substantial minority of both doctors and patients who will continue to prefer a noninstitutional setting for as much of their medical care as is possible. And I see no reason why this minority preference cannot be combined with the majority trend to institutional practice. This, it seems to me, is one of the advantages of the hospital as principal coordinator of care. Coordination does not mean swallowing up. It does not even mean physical integration. As already noted in the definition of our model, it means primarily functional and organizational relationships. And there is no technical reason—there will be political and human resistances—why the hospital cannot exercise the same qualitative and quantitative controls over its attending staff for work done in their private offices as it now exercises over them for work done on the hospital premises.

With the development of computers, it would be entirely possible to plug each physician—even the die-hard soloist—into the hospital record-keeping and retrieval system, thus overcoming one of the principal shortcomings of solo practice while retaining the very real advantages of decentralized primary care.

Fourth is the problem of authority. Where is the hospital going to get the power to do the things I have been talking about? No one knows just how this is going to evolve. But there can be no doubt that the American people are going to move toward some sort of system in the delivery and financing of health care. This system could be predominantly governmental, it could be imposed through some giant profit-oriented corporation—for example, some of the companies in the aerospace industry or through proliferation of some of the rapidly growing new proprietary hospital chains— or it could come about under the leadership of the existing voluntary hospitals and the medical profession. These, I believe, are the only possible alternatives. Personally, I prefer the latter. With all its shortcomings, I guess I feel a little like Hamlet who preferred to " . . . bear those ills we have/Than fly to others that we know not of."

If the hospitals and their boards and medical staffs and other health care institutions can pull themselves together to move resolutely and aggressively enough in the next few years, I think the necessary degree of systemization can be achieved on a voluntary pluralistic basis, with a minimum of statutory compulsion applied at certain essential strategic points—what Walter McNerney aptly calls "selective intervention." For example, the major thrust of the important Barr Committee Report[1] recommends that effective health care planning can and should be done primarily by voluntary planning bodies with ultimate authority in a state body which in turn derives strength and power from its relation to federal funding. In other words, the strength of government is applied to make sure that the voluntary bodies accept their responsibilities and do their job but it does not do the job for them unless, of course, they abdicate and refuse to do it themselves.

Similarly, with respect to physician-hospital relations, standards of physician competence, conduct, and performance should be set and enforced by peer groups based in the hospitals. The authority of government should be used only to make sure that all physicians are in fact subject to some such peer group control and that the hospitals are in fact exercising such controls in a responsible and accountable manner. Thus, I would favor compulsory affiliation of all physicians with a hospital as a condition of continued licensure.

This combination of public and private responsibility constitutes, in my view, pluralism at its best. I believe the United States Congress and most state legislatures would happily do their part to see to it that the hospitals are given the necessary authority if only the hospitals are willing to take on the job. Remember, again, when I say hospital I mean the entire institution including consumer as well as provider interests.

Finally, and in my view, the biggest of all barriers to achievement of the model is lack of vision. I agree completely that designing a theoretical model is no substitute for developing a real hospital or a real hospital system. Nevertheless, the opposite fallacy is just as bad. The world is full of good souls who simply cannot conceive of a world free of war, or free of poverty, or racial prejudice, or where medical care is provided on the basis of a rational cooperative system. Perhaps I should even add where hospital administrators, boards, and medical staff work cooperatively together for the common good!

"I have a dream," said Martin Luther King and he was correct in knowing where to start. "If you don't have a dream," said

1. United States Department of Health, Education, and Welfare, Secretary's Advisory Committee on Hospital Effectiveness, *Report*, 1968.

Bloody Mary to the young lovers in *South Pacific*, "How you gonna make a dream come true?" Or, as it is said in the Old Testament, "Without vision, the people perish." My guess is that the biggest single obstacle to achievement of the rational health care system outlined here is the general lack of conception that it is possible or what the system might look like even if all the obstacles were removed.

SIGNS OF PROGRESS

I have deliberately emphasized the obstacles because, like most pragmatists, I hate nothing worse than to be accused of wishful thinking or starry-eyed idealism. Nevertheless, as I look about the national health care scene, it seems to me there are some significant portents of progress.

I think, for example, of the many hospitals in my own state of New Jersey—often alleged to be one of the most backward in this respect—that have recently added full-time directors of medical education, that have recently staffed their emergency rooms on a full-time basis, and that have applied for grants, or are otherwise seriously considering, establishing first-class, one-class, ambulatory services in place of their traditional indigent clinics.

I think, for example, of the many neighborhood health centers that have been established throughout the country in the past three to four years. While some of these are free-standing, organizationally as well as physically—a fact that I regret—I have no doubt that eventually most of them will become satellites of hospitals.

I think, for example, of the progress of hospital planning—progress that has been temporarily confused and in some places set back by the apparently contradictory philosophy and experience of the two new planning bills—89–749 and 89–239. But progress which, almost surely, will be resumed and, hopefully, strengthened by the new laws, simply because there is no other effective way to deal with costs short of direct government control.

I think, for example, of the American Hospital Association's courageous effort to write planning and planning sanctions into the hospital reimbursement formula through its *Statement on Financial Requirements.*

59

I think, for example, of the significant Catholic Hospital Association *Statement on Comprehensive Care*, already referred to, with its strong emphasis on the role of the hospital.

Most important of all, I think of the hundreds, perhaps thousands, of individual hospitals, and other health care institutions—big and small, community and university, open staff and closed staff, rich and poor, across the country that are at this moment exploring ways in which they can relate more effectively to their communities, ways in which they can relate more effectively to the physicians and other health professionals in those communities, and ways in which they can provide better medical care to all the people in those communities.

What you are doing here today, for example, in this 19th Annual Southern Conference on Gerontology, with its focus on the effective use of health care resources, is an excellent example of what I am talking about. I congratulate Dr. Osterbind, the Institute of Gerontology, and all the participants on this impressive undertaking.

Of course what it will mean in practice depends entirely on what you do when you return to your own communities. To any of you who decide to work toward the Mercy Community Hospital model, I hardly need emphasize that it will not be an easy job. It is not a job for the timid, the tired, or the overly conservative. Nor for that matter is it for the extreme radical. You cannot hope to improve an institution—hospital, university, or any other—by destroying it.

But, increasingly, it is recognized today that the most important job of leadership—if one wishes to avoid the fate of the dinosaurs—is the engineering of social and institutional change to keep up with the scientific and technological progress. With all due respect to the laboratory scientists and engineers, I feel sure that the constructive leadership of human beings—the adaptation of human institutions—is far more difficult than the handling of bricks and mortar or even molecules.

So you who have the burden of leadership and policy-making in the health care field should have the prayers of every American as you go about this task for the lives and well-being of millions depend upon what you do or do not do. Nor will it be much comfort to remind you of Ralph Waldo Emerson's saying, "God offers to every mind its choice between truth and repose. Take which you please. You can never have both."

But there is another side to this coin. Along with the endless hours of conferences and meetings that you will have to live through, the tons of committee reports and documents that you will have to read, and the sleepless nights when you will lie awake worrying what to do next, there will, I feel sure, come the satisfaction of knowing that you are, in fact, moulding the future American health care system.

In short, to paraphrase President Roosevelt, there is not the slightest doubt in my mind that this generation of health professionals has a rendezvous with destiny!

In concluding I would like to offer one word of advice which I take from another well-known American institution. I refer to the Playboy Club of Chicago which, I am told, has the following motto engraved over its entrance in very elegant Latin script: "Si non oscillas, noli tintinari." Translated into the vernacular, this means: "Man, if you can't swing, don't ring!"

Optimum Utilization of Nursing Homes for Patient Care Needs

by DOROTHY McCAMMAN

WHAT IS MEANT by optimum utilization of nursing homes for patient care needs? First, what do we include as a nursing home? I have purposely avoided the complex, technical definitions used in licensure laws, accreditation standards, and Federal and State legislation and regulations relating to reimbursement under Medicare and public assistance programs. Instead, I am using a definition designed to be understandable to the layman —the consumer of nursing home care.

The September, 1969, issue of *Changing Times* contains an interesting article entitled "Nursing Homes: How to Pick a Good One." Three general types of nursing homes are identified in terms of the level of service provided as follows:

> *Extended-care facilities* provide continuous nursing service for convalescent patients, generally on a short-term basis, under the direction of one or more physicians. Registered nurses are backed up by licensed practical nurses and aides so that the care provided can be considered an extension of the acute care provided by a hospital.
> *Skilled-nursing homes* provide continuous nursing service, usually on a long-term basis, under the direction of a registered professional nurse. A good skilled-nursing home will

have advisory physicians who review the home's program and advise on its medical problems.

Residential or intermediate-care homes provide regular and frequent medical and nursing services, in addition to room and board, for persons not capable of fully independent living. In the best intermediate-care homes, a registered professional nurse is the supervisor of nursing. At the very least, care should be under the supervision of a licensed practical nurse.

Because our concern is with patient care, the definitions most useful for my purpose are those of extended care facilities and skilled nursing homes.

What then do we mean by optimum? An old edition of Webster's International Unabridged offers this definition: The best or most favorable degree, quantity, etc. Best or most favorable from whose point of view? The patient, the doctor, the nursing home, the taxpayer? A more recent Webster's Collegiate is somewhat more helpful: The amount or degree of something that is most favorable to some end. Since we are talking about patient care needs, some end can then be interpreted as the betterment of the patient. But we are still faced with questions of how to measure the amount or degree that is most favorable and who makes the determination.

Under present circumstances—and I hasten to say that these are not optimum—the major determinant of the amount and degree of nursing home utilization can be said to be the amount of public funds made available to pay for nursing home care. Public funds also determine the amount of community services which if more widely available could often eliminate the need for institutionalization.

Currently, about three out of every four dollars expended for nursing home care come from public sources. In the fiscal year ended in 1969, expenditures for nursing home care totalled $2.4 billion, or 4 per cent of the aggregate personal health care expenditures for the nation. That the public stake is especially great in relation to nursing homes is clear from the fact that just over one-third (35.6 per cent) of all personal health care finances—$60.3 billion in fiscal 1969—is publicly financed.

Of the $1.8 billion in public monies that went to nursing homes in that year, $400 million was through the Medicare program. A far larger amount—nearly $1.4 billion—was through federal-state programs of public assistance. The remainder of about $41 million was paid under Veterans programs.

The Social Security Administration's series on health expenditures throws light on the increasing importance of nursing homes in the health care dollar, and especially the public dollar. Back in 1950, nursing home care amounted to $142 million, claiming just over 1 per cent of all national health expenditures; and for every dollar of government expenditures for nursing home care, nearly four came out of private pockets. By 1960, the proportion of all health expenditures going to nursing homes had reached 2 per cent and the ratio of private to public was still nearly four to one.

During the 1960's, public expenditures for nursing homes climbed at a considerably faster rate than did private expenditures, and in 1966—the last year before Medicare entered into the extended care field—$1.00 in government money was spent for every $1.20 in private. The dramatic reversal in this ratio came in 1967. Private expenditures for nursing home care decreased slightly and public expenditures almost doubled, with the result that close to $2 was spent under public programs for every $1 from private funds.

Not all of these national expenditures for nursing home care are spent on behalf of the aged. But the aged account for such a preponderant share of all nursing home costs that the above summary adequately reflects the trend over the years if one is concerned only with these costs for the aged. For recent years, estimates developed by the Social Security Administration permit separate consideration of health expenditures for the population sixty-five years and over.

In fiscal year 1968, total personal health care expenditures for the aged amounted to $11.4 billion, a medical bill of $590.40 per aged person. Of this total, 30 per cent was paid privately and 70 per cent publicly. Included were nursing-home care expenditures that totalled $1.8 billion, or $91.28 per capita if spread evenly over the population sixty-five and older—and they most obviously are not spread evenly. Of the nursing home care expenditures, 22.7 per cent came from private sources, a drastic drop from the preceding fiscal year when the private portion had been 46.1 per cent. Medicare paid 18.7 per cent of the nursing home costs for the aged, leaving 58.6 per cent for Medicaid and other public programs.

Reflecting the greater availability of public funds and the accompanying rise in nursing homes and related facilities, the proportion of the aged population resident in these facilities increased almost four-fold from 1954 to 1967—from 1.1 per cent to 3.6 per cent—as estimated by the Department of Health, Education, and Welfare. Clearly then, public financing is now playing and will continue to play a major role in determining the amount and degree of nursing home care. No one would claim that the role played thus far has produced optimum utilization, however defined.

A very simple definition of optimum utilization of health services is "the right patient in the right bed at the right time—or not in bed at all." This is a medical determination but it has clear-cut implications for the purchaser of services too because frequently the most appropriate level of care is also the most economical. In comparison to hospital rates that are approaching $100 a day, care in an extended care facility that costs $35 a day or in a skilled-nursing home at $20–$25 a day may be optimum from both points of view, but not when the patient's welfare could be better served by a home health program that made institutional care unnecessary in the first place or that shortened the stay. And not when timely health screening and preventive services could reduce illness and the need for medical care.

To say that optimum utilization of nursing homes is a medical determination is an oversimplification. Suppose a doctor prescribes a nursing home as optimum and a nursing home bed is not available, necessitating a hospital stay longer than medically indicated or premature discharge to the patient's home, whether or not home health services are available? Suppose the only nursing home beds are way out in the country, inaccessible to relatives and friends who could contribute to the patient's social well-being and to the doctor who is essential to his physical well-being? Or that the aged patient with limited financial resources has insurance that would cover his hospitalization but not his nursing home care?

Let's look then at the barriers to optimum utilization of nursing homes for patient care needs. The first barrier to the optimum use

65

of nursing homes is the unavailability of the most appropriate service in the continuum of health care. This cuts both ways: it encompasses the underuse of a nursing home by a patient who is unnecessarily in an expensive short-term hospital, as well as the overuse by a patient whose recovery would be facilitated by a program of care in his own home.

Until the full range of alternative health services is uniformly available—and by available I mean not only developed but financially available—patient care is bound to be less than optimum, not just in nursing homes but in other health facilities too.

As an example of the overuse of nursing homes, I would call attention to a 1960 report of a study by the Illinois Public Aid Commission which concluded that nearly half of all persons now served in skilled nursing homes could be at home if they had welcoming families, or in boarding homes if minimum additional care were provided.

And as an example of the overuse of hospitals, let me cite from testimony presented to our Committee's Subcommittee on Health of the Elderly during 1967 hearings on Costs and Delivery of Health Services to Older Americans. The testimony of the Community Council of Greater New York included the following quotations from a letter sent by a hospital in New York City which was described as typical:

Over one thousand extra days of hospital care were necessary during a period of eight months because of lack of facilities in the community to provide nursing home, chronic care and home help for patients 65 and over, in this institution.

It was possible in some instances to send patients home with homemakers and various types of home help. In one instance which is typical of many, patient was sent home after waiting 26 days for admission into a nursing home. There was a problem in obtaining the needed services and special funds had to be used to meet cost until a voluntary homemaker agency could meet the need. If Home Help had been more readily available, patient could have been sent home earlier.

It is also of interest to note that many patients do so well, at home when there is help, often to an unanticipated degree that applications for nursing home care have often been cancelled. . . .

Too often nursing home care has been planned only because nothing else was available. This has seemingly resulted in a poor use of nursing home facilities.[1]

No one—to the best of my knowledge—has developed a blueprint that would spell out the number of beds of different types that would be required to provide optimum nursing home care in the continuum of health services. A look at the data on the number of beds per 1,000 Medicare enrollees in participating extended care facilities makes all too clear the wide disparity that now exists. On July 31, 1968, the number of beds per 1,000 Medicare enrollees in the United States was 17.1 and the range was from 41.6 in Connecticut to 4.6 in Mississippi (Florida, incidentally, was 15.6; Georgia, 17.3; South Carolina, 17.8; and North Carolina, 8.2). All too clearly, whatever the optimum is, a tenfold range in the ratio leaves entirely too much room for any reasonable geographical difference.

Clearly, the optimum will vary depending on what other facilities are within the geographic and financial reach of the patient. Even when financial barriers are eliminated in relation to the full continuum of health services, there may be very different levels of utilization of nursing home services depending primarily on how these services are integrated. I would cite as an example, two projects financed by the United States Public Health Service to provide extended care facility services and home health benefits to members of prepaid group health plans who were below age sixty-five. One of these group health plans owned its own hospital, had just completed an adjacent extended care facility attached to the hospital, and with the advent of Medicare, had organized its own home care agency—all physically integrated into the central hospital complex and a time-tested medical care system. The other plan used the community hospitals that had long provided care for their members, with Blue Cross as an intermediary, and, to carry out the project, contracted with two extended care facilities and with the home health programs of the visiting nurse service and

---

1. U.S. Senate Special Committee on Aging, Hearings of the Subcommittee on Health of the Elderly, *Costs and Delivery of Health Services to Older Americans*, 90th Cong., 1st sess., October, 1967, Part 2, p. 455.

of a hospital that had received national recognition for its rehabilitation achievements with the aged.

Both plans significantly reduced hospital utilization, even though the first of these two was already at what had been thought to be rock-bottom utilization and the other was well below the national average. But in the first plan, the use of an extended care facility integrated into the hospital complex—at an average cost per day of $35.40—almost balanced the decrease in acute hospital days; not many hospital days were saved by admissions to the home-care services. In the second group health plan, very little use was made of the extended care facilities—remember, this is an under sixty-five population—and hospital stays were shortened or made unnecessary through the use of home health services which, although provided by local agencies, were stimulated and used imaginatively by the plan's coordinator, a registered nurse. Utilization of nursing home care, while dramatically different under the two projects, was probably optimum considering the way in which the plans were organized to deliver the continuum of health services.

Without doubt, a major barrier to the optimum utilization of nursing homes—resulting in the overuse of hospitals—has been the fact that Blue Cross and other private health insurance programs were organized to meet the costs of care in hospitals rather than in nursing homes or other lesser care facilities. Under Medicare too, the primary purpose was to relieve the aged of the most devastating costs of hospitalization. Extended care and home health services were included in order to prevent the overutilization of hospitals, not because they offered a better and more suitable way of meeting the older person's medical care needs.

Appropriate to this purpose then, Medicare limits the coverage for care in extended care facilities to patients who have been in the hospital for three days or longer and enter the facility within fourteen days after leaving the hospital.

Has the three-day requirement served to prevent over-utilization of hospitals or has it instead increased hospital costs through unnecessary admissions solely to qualify for the extended care benefit? No purpose is served here by debating this question. The fact remains that the three-day requirement hinders achievement of optimum utilization of *both* hospitals and nursing homes. The requirement also poses a serious problem of medical ethics. Again quoting from the hearings on Costs and Delivery of Health Services, a doctor introduced an article from *Medical Economics* entitled "Medical Ethics and Medicare" and illustrated the problem in relation to a patient who has a chronic urinary tract infection:

> This man should be in a nursing home. The nursing home will charge for, we will say, 2 weeks or something like that. At any rate, the total bill for the nursing home would be $1,400.
>
> Now if he admits that patient to the hospital for 3 days or whatever the minimum requirement is, he can then transfer the patient to the nursing home and instead of paying $1,400 the patient pays $400.
>
> In other words, by admitting this patient to the hospital for a workup which is not really necessary but which could be medically justified, he will save the patient $1,000.
>
> Now in a situation like that what do you do? Do you admit the patient for 3 or 4 days of hospitalization so you can save him $1,000 or do you send him directly to the nursing facility?
>
> These are tough questions in medical ethics.[2]

And the doctor goes on to say: "Now, again, what is optimum care? Here it is pretty difficult to define. If you give him 2 extra days, is this bad medical care, is that a lowering of your standards? It is difficult to define it. I think the medical profession generally, if the money is not coming out of the patient's pocket, tends to give a little more hospitalization, a little more medicine, a little more everything else."[3]

The level of payment is undoubtedly another major barrier to optimum development and utilization of nursing homes. Unfortunately, this country has a long and well-established tradition of underpayment by the government for the health services it purchases. Especially for nursing homes where perhaps half or more of all patients in recent years have had at least part of their costs paid by welfare. This tradition has hampered the development of the high quality care implicit in optimum utilization.

The old question of which came first the chicken or the egg?

2. *Ibid.*, Part 1, p. 42.
3. *Ibid.*, p. 46.

was brought forcibly to my attention when I participated in a survey of aging programs in a New England State back in the mid-fifties. In application, the question was simply this: can the Welfare Department raise its payment to nursing homes to encourage the provision of rehabilitation services before these services actually exist? And can nursing homes afford to introduce such services before the cash is on the barrelhead?

About this same time—and this was in a period when at least one southern state had a maximum payment of about $1 a day for an Old-Age Assistance recipient, whether or not in a nursing home —the Illinois Public Aid Commission embarked upon a geriatrics rehabilitation program to demonstrate the potentials for restoring nursing home patients to independent living. This project, carried out on a demonstration basis in Peoria and Cook County, provided for financing the cost of medical and social rehabilitation services for public assistance recipients in nursing homes. It produced clearcut evidence that many old-age assistance recipients could be restored to independent living instead of spending their remaining days in a nursing home or mental hospital. Many of those who were enabled to live at home no longer needed public aid or needed far less than the cost of care in a nursing home or hospital. In fact, the savings in public assistance payments for the first year alone were about equal to the cost of the project.

The success of the demonstration caused the Illinois Public Aid Commission to build into its assistance rates on a continuing basis an incentive payment on behalf of assistance recipients in nursing homes with approved rehabilitation programs; the differential consisted of a higher rate of payment made across-the-board for all public assistance recipients in the nursing home plus an additional amount for the individual for whom the home has a specific rehabilitation program prescribed by the doctor.

The Washington State Public Assistance Agency several years later introduced a rehabilitation program modeled on that of Illinois. One large county in another state experimented with the use of a supplementary payment by the health department to encourage the provision of rehabilitation services for assistance recipients in nursing homes.

But, to the best of my knowledge, these scattered efforts have had relatively little national impact over the years. Even in Peoria, Illinois—the pioneer—which I had occasion to study in the mid-1960's while working on a Brandeis University–Ford Foundation project, only a few nursing homes were currently approved for differential payments.

Why haven't such efforts been more widespread, in view of their demonstrable success? I suspect that part of the answer lies in the attitude of the operators of nursing homes who, by and large, would prefer not to take welfare patients at all and who find it more profitable to keep a patient in bed once admitted, instead of embarking on a program of rehabilitation and then releasing him. When the Illinois Public Aid Commission rehabilitation project was first announced, the operators of local nursing homes rose up in indignation over what they thought was an effort to drive them out of business. Staff responsible for the project argued diligently to persuade the nursing homes to cooperate. As the project developed, however, resistance was reduced because the operators could see the business value of services that maximize the recovery potential of the patient; staff members were easier to recruit and keep because they found satisfaction in serving human beings rather than vegetables. It was clear that even if rehabilitation achieves its maximum potential, there will continue to be plenty of older people whose optimum care is in a nursing home of high quality.

The fact remains that public assistance programs as a whole do not pay rates that would encourage acceptance of welfare patients, to say nothing of rates that cover the extra costs of rehabilitation and restorative services. And regardless of who pays, there is no incentive to reduce the costs of administration and management or to discharge patients promptly.

What *does* welfare pay for nursing home costs? Costs, according to the *Changing Times* article mentioned earlier, are likely to start at $350 to $500 a month for a semi-private room and $500 to $800 for a private room as *basic* charges, with the certainty that there will always be extra charges of uncertain amount.

And here I quote from unpublished testimony taken at the July 30, 1969, hearing of the United States Senate Subcommittee on Long-Term Care. The statement of the American Nursing Homes

Health Care Services for the Aged

Association (ANHA) included the following summary of per diem rates paid for skilled nursing home care under Medicaid or other public assistance programs in states that had not yet adopted Medicaid: "As of January 1, 1969, maximum per diem rates for maximum care ranged from a low of $4 to a high of slightly over $20 per day among the 43 States responding to the survey. A majority of the reporting States, 24 to be exact, have a maximum rate of $10 per day or less for maximum care, including room, board and nursing services. But the average payment per patient day actually made by State agencies was $7 or less in 25 States and $10 or less in 40 of the 43 States reporting. And, in fact, 12 States pay less than the cost of care and are forced to encourage supplementation payments from families and local subdivisions to finance skilled nursing home care.

"The survey, conducted by ANHA among the State welfare agencies, also showed that while 25 States had increased payments between January 1, 1968 and January 1, 1969, five actually had decreased payments and 13 had retained maximum payments at the same levels despite the obvious increase in the cost of care over the preceding year."

As barriers to the optimum use of nursing homes, I have flagged first the lack of more suitable health services, or organizational and financing patterns that deter the use of these alternatives, and second the lack of the financial incentives (particularly through public payments) that would assure optimum care.

There are other barriers. One of these is the lack of information about where to find a good nursing home and how to judge the quality of a home. Some months ago, *Parade,* appearing in many of our Sunday newspapers, carried a story on nursing homes. As a source of information about good nursing homes, it cited the National Council of Senior Citizens. This organization had no advance warning that its name would appear in the story and it makes no pretense of keeping abreast on the subject of nursing homes. In the week following the story, the National Council of Senior Citizens received nearly 1,000 letters pleading for the names of good nursing homes in areas clear across the country.

In all too many cases, the selection of a nursing home must be made on an emergency basis—one just pushes the panic button.

72

The *Changing Times* article to which I have already referred contains a number of excellent yardsticks for use in selecting the type of nursing home and level of care most suited to the patient's needs. Unfortunately, it gives insufficient recognition to the fact that the level of care needed may shift, sometimes from day to day but almost inevitably as the years go by. And it virtually dooms to failure the search for a good skilled nursing home or extended care facility by singling out as the one characteristic that matters most: Is this a happy place? Hospitals are not happy places. Extended care facilities that truly meet their objective of shortening the hospital stay and rehabilitating the patient are not designed primarily to be happy places. Nursing homes that offer skilled nursing care *should be* much pleasanter and happier than most of them are, and certainly a residential or personal care home should make every effort to provide a happy environment for its residents.

Perhaps in this lies a clue to the means for achieving optimum nursing home utilization for *patient care.* There is still entirely too much confusion about the proper role of nursing homes in providing the optimum level of patient care.

Nursing homes are in transition. They are no longer merely a place to die. The traditional view of a nursing home as a long-term terminal-care facility is outmoded. Their new role is a sort of way station between the hospital and the home, and the term home includes a variety of living arrangements ranging from the older person's own home where supportive services make possible independent living to residential or personal care homes for the aged.

Medicare, while providing an opportunity to maximize this new role through its extended care benefits, has added to this confusion. To too many people, the term extended care has meant, and still means, long drawn out care rather than post-hospital convalescent care. The confusion was compounded when the interpretation of participating extended care facilities which is permitted under Medicare opened the door to skilled nursing homes that were never designed, and could not be redesigned, to provide the level of patient care implicit in the concept of extended care.

On this point, I turn to the St. Petersburg hearings held by the Senate Committee's Subcommittee on Long-Term Care on January 9, 1970, and specifically to the expert testimony of Charles W.

Pruitt, Jr., Executive Director of the Cathedral Foundation of Jacksonville, who said: "Extended care as a level of care cannot and was probably never intended to be provided in the typical nursing home. Specifically designed and equipped facilities will be constructed to provide this level of care and most will be attached to or closely related to general hospitals.

"The unfortunate interpretation of extended care which was allowed under Medicare when it was initiated permitted most nursing homes to attempt to provide this level of care. This decision will haunt us for several years and will cause continued misunderstanding of the term. However, extended care, in its true sense, will flourish in the Seventies and bring about its potential of better and more economical patient care. The attitudes of health administrators and physicians in both hospitals and nursing homes toward the extended-care concept will be the determinant factor in how quickly the community can benefit."

Mr. Pruitt went on to predict that the seventies will see the rise of the voluntary nonprofit sponsor as the dominant force in the long-term care field. He summarized the factors that will bring about this change from proprietary dominance—nearly two-thirds of the nation's licensed nursing home beds are now in proprietary homes—as follows: "Community health planning, higher standards for licensure and accreditation, development of health personnel standards by professional groups, the entry of increasing numbers of hospitals into the long-term care field, the public's demand for quality service at the lowest possible cost, and the growing number of housing-for-the-elderly projects sponsored by non-profit groups."

As a health economist concerned primarily that high quality care be available through the most economical method, I wholeheartedly endorse Mr. Pruitt's expert analysis. We are now at the crossroads and he presents compelling reasons for taking the voluntary nonprofit road.

Optimum utilization of nursing homes cannot be achieved without higher standards of construction and staffing. These higher standards are increasingly difficult for proprietary facilities to meet if they are to maintain the profit ratio demanded by owners and by the ever larger number of investors in nursing homes.

The nursing home business has become an ever bigger business but I do not think that the avenue to their optimum use is through the "Big Board" of the Stock Exchange. Let me read to you from the January 15, 1970, Research Department Weekly Bulletin of a stock brokerage firm with which I am familiar: "Another of last year's strong groups, the nursing home–medical services concept, has turned quite mixed. Although far from a mature industry, many of the companies have now been in existence long enough to permit keener analytical observations, involving greater depth value of management capabilities, plans, accounting procedures, and financial stability. *To some degree, the market is tending to separate the men from the boys*" (emphasis added).

If these are the criteria that determine success or failure—criteria related only to profit and business acumen, completely without consideration of the consumer's interest—any profits to be gained go to the investor who picks the right chain, not to the nursing home patient.

Similarly, less newsworthy efforts to capitalize on the *business* of providing nursing home care have too often resulted in profits for the owners rather than the consumers. During the recent St. Petersburg hearing, a major witness referred to the trend toward combining homes under single ownership in order to take advantage of volume purchasing, volume management and hopefully volume profit. With respect to this trend, he commented: "These homes in the St. Petersburg area which utilize that concept, however, upon investigation reveal a slightly lower level of service than other homes in the same area." We might ask if this lower level is coincidental or instead the inevitable result of a competitive business run on the profit motive.

The operators of nursing homes are not alone in the blame for failure to achieve high levels of extended care. Why should they reduce their profits in order to develop a program of patient care that the consumer has not yet learned to demand and that is not yet even accepted by many physicians?

Community health planning, which Mr. Pruitt includes as one of the factors that will result in growing community support for nonprofit facilities, will hopefully result in the availability of the full range of health facilities and services that make possible optimum use of nursing homes. One must recognize, however, that the focus of community planning in the past by health professionals has been on the hospital and the acute care it provides. There must be a concerted effort by consumers to assure that today's planning takes into account the continuum of health services needed for patient care including preventive as well as rehabilitative services.

Hospitals, primarily under voluntary, nonprofit sponsorship, are increasingly accepting responsibility for providing broader community health services involving the operation of long-term care and related facilities, either as integral organizational parts of the hospital or as attached facilities. In this trend lies a bright hope for optimum utilization of nursing homes for patient care. Hospital affiliation (and I mean more than just the affiliation agreements between hospitals and nursing homes that are required by Medicare, too many of which exist on paper only) makes possible a coordinated medical care program under the supervision of the teaching hospital. The patient and his needs are paramount, not the facility in which he happens to be located at the moment. Integration of health facilities requires that nursing homes and other facilities give up their autonomy and become cooperative rather than competitive. It is hard to see the usual proprietary nursing home in this non-autonomous role, particularly in view of its past history of reluctance to use rehabilitation, dietary and visiting nurse services that have long been available on a cooperative basis from community agencies. Some nursing homes would resist the medical supervision that is part of hospital affiliation. When I was working on the Brandeis project, one nursing home operator told me with pride that the doctors of his patients trusted the home to provide any necessary medical services—that over 75 per cent of their business with doctors was transacted over the phone. He said —and I quote him verbatim—"We give the diagnosis to them over the phone, and they prescribe and send out medication." No one could call this optimum nursing home utilization for patient care.

In this paper, I have perhaps overemphasized what is *not* optimum. This is almost inevitable since I draw my examples primarily from the recent past and from the existing situation. And at present, the situation is far from optimum. I believe, however, that we are now ready to put into action the lessons we have learned about long-term care in the context of total community health.

Knowledge, Need, and Use of Services Among the Aged

by FLOYD J. FOWLER, JR.

THE MAIN PURPOSE of the project discussed in this paper is to identify factors that account for why aged people for whom services are appropriate do not make use of them.[1] In looking for a general pattern, a range of services were included in the project: homemaker services, home nursing services, counseling, vocational assistance, and the Golden Age Club program. Because the focus of this conference is health-related services, this paper will concentrate on the home nursing service. However, our conclusions are also based on the data concerning the other services, particularly homemaker service and social clubs for the aged, and occasionally I shall refer to those data as well.

Two central conclusions have arisen from our research. First, the demographic groups among the aged at whom services are most clearly aimed are least likely to seek, and hence receive, service. Second, the most important single factor in under-utilization is lack of knowledge about the service system. In the balance of this paper, I shall outline the bases for these conclusions and some of their implications.

1. The analysis was supported jointly by the Combined Jewish Philanthropies of Greater Boston and also by Administration on Aging Grant No. AA-4-68-024-03.

Design

The research was based on a survey study of the aged (those sixty-five or older) living in metropolitan Boston. An area probability sample of all housing units in the Standard Metropolitan Statistical Area was drawn. Over 6,000 addresses were screened, and interviews averaging just less than an hour in length were taken when an aged person was located. The result was a sample of 1,350 aged persons.[2]

The questionnaire covered a variety of topics including considerable demographic information, information about health and leisure time activities, as well as information about services. The questions on services followed a generally consistent pattern:

(1) Would you know of a (GIVEN SERVICE)?

(2) Have you ever needed this kind of help?

(3) And did you get the help?

The services were described to respondents as follows:

(1) A service "set up to help people in getting a job or getting retraining for another job."

(2) A service "where a person could get a nurse to help out a person who is ill at home."

(3) A service "where you can get someone to help out around the house when the housewife is ill."

(4) An agency "set up to help someone with a family or personal problem."

We also asked whether the respondent knew of any "special activities or organizations for people over 60" and whether he had ever participated in such activities.

Use of Services

Our first step in the analysis was to see who reported needing and using services. We particularly looked at need for and use of home nursing service, in part because the rate of reported need

2. The response rate was 70 per cent. This is lower than our normal response rate. The main reason was that a Bureau of the Budget delay necessitated a three-month lag between the screening and the interviewing, during which time some selected respondents moved or died.

was highest for that of all the services we asked about. We selected six groups for special attention. We looked at those who reported at least two chronic health conditions or who rated their health fair or poor because their rate of need for home nursing should have been relatively high. We looked at the less educated, those with low incomes, and immigrants because we thought they were groups that community agencies particularly aimed to serve. Also, our data, like others, showed a higher incidence of health problems among the poor and less educated.[3] Finally, we looked at those seventy-five and older, both because they have relatively poor health and relatively fewer private resources than other aged people.

TABLE 1

PERCENTAGE WHO REPORT NEVER NEEDING HOME NURSING
SERVICE BY EDUCATION

EDUCATION	PERCENTAGE NEVER NEEDING
Less than 9 grades	84
9–11 grades	85
High school graduation	82
Some college or more	72

The basic relationships that emerged from this initial step set the course for all our further work. Briefly stated, only one of our target groups reported significantly higher need for or use of home nursing service than others. Those who had two or more chronic health conditions reported more need for and use of home nursing service than those with one or two health conditions. However, the young aged and the older aged, those who rated their health as good and those who rated their health as fair or poor, immigrants and native-born Americans all reported very comparable rates of need and use. The most striking relationship was that those who had attended college reported significantly more need for and use of home nursing than those who were less educated. There was also a significant trend for the aged with the lowest incomes to report less need and use of home nursing services.

3. E.g. "Medical Care, Health Status, and Family Income," *Vital and Health Statistics* (Washington: United States Department of Health, Education, and Welfare, Public Health Service, 1964), Series 10, Number 9.

Health Care Services for the Aged

Note that it was not simply reported rates of service utilization that showed this pattern. It was also the rates of reported need. Thus it was not simply that our proposed need groups were not getting home nursing service. It was also the case that they did not think they needed this service. Generally comparable patterns emerged with respect to homemaker service, and the rates of reported use of social clubs for the aged showed a similar discrepancy between our expectations about whom they are designed to serve and who reported using them. Moreover, in each case the better

TABLE 2

PERCENTAGE WHO REPORT NEVER NEEDING HOME NURSING SERVICE BY TOTAL ANNUAL FAMILY INCOME

TOTAL ANNUAL FAMILY INCOME	PERCENTAGE NEVER NEEDING
Less than $2000	87
$2000–$3999	83
$4000–$5999	80
$6000 or over	78

educated reported more need and use of services than the less educated. It was these education relationships which led us to focus our attention on the role of knowledge.

KNOWLEDGE ABOUT SERVICES

One sure way a survey researcher can evoke a surprised response from a sophisticated audience is to report the percentage of a population that possesses a given bit of presumably common knowledge. On almost any topic, public information is at a lower level than most people suppose. In this respect, the information level of the aged in greater Boston about services is no exception. The key question was: Do you know whether there is any service in the community, or convenient to you, where a person could get a nurse to help out a person who is ill at home? Note that to say yes to this question, a person did not need to know the name of the agency or its location—only that there was a program like this in the community. Thus, the question represents a minimum test of information, but it is the criterion we shall use when we say a person knew of a service.

Forty-five per cent of the greater Boston aged knew of the home nursing program, which is also to say that about 55 per cent did not know of the program. About the same percentage knew of Golden Age activities. The rest of the services we asked about were much less known. Less than a quarter knew of homemaker services, employment services, or family counseling services.

Knowledge about each service, like most measures of information, was highly related to level of education. While overall close to half said they know about a home nursing service, two-thirds of

TABLE 3

PERCENTAGE WHO REPORT KNOWING ABOUT VARIOUS SERVICES

TYPE OF SERVICE	PERCENTAGE KNOWING
Home nursing	46
Homemaker	14
General counseling	22
Employment	24
Golden Age clubs	49

those who had been to college knew about such a service compared with only one-third of those who had not gone beyond the eighth grade. All of the target groups discussed earlier—those over age seventy-five, immigrants, those with low incomes, and those in poorer health—generally have less education and they are, as a result, less knowledgeable than average about services.

We have thus far established three points. First, our target groups report use of home nursing at the same or lower rates than others. Second, with one exception, they are no more likely, and particularly in the cases of the poor and the less educated, less likely, than other aged to think they have ever needed this service. Third, they are less likely to know about this service. The question is whether there is a relationship between the level of information a person has about a service and the likelihood of his perceiving a need for that service.

Two Models

There are at least two models one can posit about a relationship between need for a service and knowledge about a service. These models are generally not explicit, but I believe the most commonly assumed model goes something like this. A person first sees that he has a problem with which he needs help. If he knows where help is available, he seeks it. If he does not know, he seeks information about sources of help for his problem. I think we tend to think of the breakdown in service delivery as occurring at the service-seeking level. The person cannot find the right agency, he is not eligible, he refuses to accept agency help, expenses are a barrier, and so on. In this model, the perception of need may precede obtaining information about the kinds of services available.

This model probably is quite appropriate for some kinds of problems. The examples that come to mind are those in which the problem is too severe to be ignored and the nature of the problem is unambiguous. Thus severe acute medical conditions, injuries, and out-of-wedlock pregnancies will probably lead to some help-seeking. The questions relate to where help will be sought and which kind of help will be received.

There is a second model which differs slightly but significantly from the preceding. Once again we start with a person who has a problem. If he knows about a service that helps people with this type of problem, he may decide he has a problem with which he needs help. However, if he has never heard of anyone being helped with a problem like his, he never will decide that he has a need for help or for service—he just has a problem. If he never decides he needs help, he will not pursue the task of finding out what sources of help might be available. In this second model, knowing something about services is the precondition rather than the result of knowing one needs service.

This model seems most appropriate for problems which people, in some way, can live with and for problems for which the existence and character of available service is not widely known. It seems to me that as we are more and more concerned, as a society, with not merely keeping people alive but also with making life better for them, this model will become increasingly relevant. We are starting to try to help people, particularly the aged, with problems we have never before helped them with. If this model is accurate, we are going to have to increase people's sophistication about available services in order for them to be able to know when they have a need for service.

KNOWLEDGE AND USE

Let me now present the evidence that led us to think this model is an appropriate one. Gurin *et al*[4] did a survey study of mental health in the American population. One of their clear findings was that better educated people were much more likely to seek mental health services. Their analysis points out that it requires a certain amount of sophistication to "diagnose" a problem in mental health terms. If an individual does not have this sophistica-

TABLE 4

NEED FOR THE FOUR SERVICES BY KNOWLEDGE OF THOSE
SERVICES

KNOWLEDGE OF SERVICE	NEED FOR SERVICES				
	Ever needed	Never needed	NA	Total	N
Employment Service					
Knows of service	11%	89	a	100%	(305)
Does not know					
of service	3%	97	a	100%	(998)
Home Nursing Service					
Knows of service	26%	74	a	100%	(611)
Does not know					
of service	8%	91	2	100%	(711)
Homemaker Service					
Knows of service	10%	89	1	100%	(189)
Does not know					
of service	7%	93	a	100%	(1129)
General Counseling Service					
Knows of service	6%	93	1	100%	(294)
Does not know					
of service	2%	98	a	100%	(1017)

a. Less than 0.5 per cent

tion, including some information about mental health services, he will never code a problem as indicating a need for psychiatric help.

The analysis presented previously in this paper parallels the Gurin data and can be interpreted in the same way. However, we were also able to examine these ideas, and some alternatives, in a more direct way. If our analysis is correct, those who know about a

4. Gerald Gurin, *et al.*, *Americans View Their Mental Health* (New York: Basic Books, 1960).

service should be considerably more likely to report needing a service than those who do not know about it. Remember that the "not-knowers" include disproportionate numbers of the poor, the less educated, and the very old, as well as proportionate numbers of people in poor health. So the risk factor should be working in the direction of higher need among those who do not know about the service.

The results are rather striking. Over one-fourth of all those who knew about a home nursing service reported having needed it, compared with less than 10 per cent of those who did not know about the service. In all four services studied, the same relationship was observed; three of the four were statistically significant at the .001 level of confidence. In general, those who knew about a service were two or three times as likely to report needing the service as those who did not know about it.

This seemed rather strong support for the idea that knowing something about a service is a considerable asset in recognizing a need for a service, but an alternative hypothesis was possible. Perhaps those people among the poor and the rest of the target groups who needed the service had found out about it. Hence, the knowers would consist of the better educated plus those from the rest of the population who had reason to acquire information about home nursing service. This approach would not explain the distribution of reported need, but might explain the relationship between knowledge and need. In any case, we controlled for level of education and looked for some indication that our target groups were better informed than others—some indication that the needy groups were seeking information. We found no such evidence, however. With one exception, the target groups were equally as or less informed than others, even with education controlled.[5] Thus, to us, at least, the evidence seemed compelling that some information about home nursing service, and probably other services, is a very important, if not necessary, condition for a person to recognize that he has a need for a service.

5. The exception was again those people who reported two or more chronic conditions. They were also the exception in that they were the only target group that reported relatively high need for home nursing service.

PATTERNS OF USE AMONG KNOWERS

Finally we wondered whether or not our target groups would report more need than others if we looked only at the more knowledgeable part of the population. The fact that our measure of sophistication—knowing about home nursing service—was rather crude no doubt limited the findings. The inadequacy of the measure as a control is apparent from the fact that college-educated aged and those with high incomes still generally reported more need than others even among those who know about the service. Clearly there is more to sophistication than simply having heard of home nursing. Nevertheless, there were some interesting findings.

In all cases, if one looks only at the population that knows about the service, the target groups expressed more need for the service relative to others than they did without the control. Thus, age was unrelated to reported need for all aged; but among those who knew about home nursing service, those over seventy-five report significantly more need for the service than those who are sixty-five to seventy. Among all aged, immigrants report significantly less need, but among those who know about the service, immigrants report more need. Also, although the college-educated report a high rate of need, among those who did not go to college, those with grade school only report more need than high school graduates when knowledge is controlled. Similar kinds of patterns were found in our analysis of use of social clubs for the aged. Although not definitive, these results with our rough index of sophistication are sufficient to convince us that the patterns of reported need and use of services among aged would correspond much more closely to actual need if knowledge about services were more equitably distributed.

CONCLUSIONS

At this point, some discussion of the implications of these data is in order. However, I want to dwell for a moment on two aspects of the dynamics of service-getting which were mentioned, but not developed.

First, let me go back to the one consistent exception in the data.

We have said that those who rated their health as fair or poor, those who were immigrants, very old, poor, or less educated fit our general pattern. They are using services at a lower rate relative to the total aged population than one would expect. They also report relatively less need for home nursing service when it is described to them. They have less knowledge about services than others. And finally, their rate of reported need for service increases relatively more than others when we look only at those among them who know something about services. This pattern does not fit one group, those who report having at least two chronic health conditions. This group alone of the target groups we focussed on reports relatively more need, and more use of home nursing service; and this group alone is more knowledgeable about home nursing service than average. There are a variety of explanations possible for this exception, but I tend to think about it primarily in the following terms.

The model I have outlined, that some knowledge or sophistication is a necessary or at least important condition for knowing one needs a service, applies best to those problems that one can, in some sense, live with. If the situation becomes desperate enough, I presume that the other model will apply; that the existence of a problem will lead to finding out about sources of help and to seeking that help. My own guess is that many of those reporting two or more conditions have been sick enough at some time that they could not ignore the fact that they needed help. It also seems likely that in connection with their illnesses, they were in contact with people, like doctors and other professionals at hospitals, who helped them diagnose their situation as a need for service and also provided them with some information about the resources available.

Unfortunately from a service delivery point of view, though fortunately in other respects, we are not merely interested in providing services to those in very serious condition. We are interested in helping aged through short-term problem situations; we are interested in helping with problems before they become so serious that institutionalization of one sort or another becomes the only alternative; we are interested in making life comfortable, not in simply keeping it from being intolerable. It is with respect to those problems which are very serious but less than intolerable to which I think the comments in this paper apply most directly.

A second point I want to emphasize is the fact that it seems to me that our service system places primary responsibility on the individual himself for seeking and getting the help he needs. One study we did of an agency (that may or may not be typical) indicated that well over half the clients were self-referrals; that is, they walked in or called because they had decided on their own that they needed the kind of help the agency gave. Our analysis suggests that this reliance on the individual to diagnose his own problem systematically discriminates against the least educated and others who are less able to identify their problems. Now it is true that most agencies and service programs have more requests for service than they can meet. To the extent that one can generalize rates from our data, the demand for service might be increased by 50 per cent if all aged were as informed as our group of knowers. Indeed this may be an underestimate, as it appears that those who do not know about services may have a higher incidence of real need for service than those who know about services. However, the present system appears to select people on an irrelevant basis —the fact that they do not know enough to seek service. A better system would have professionals making the decisions about who has the greatest need for service.

I believe these findings on the likely relationship between knowledge and obtaining service have some very direct practical implications for at least four reasons: (1) there is such a very large relationship between knowledge and perceived need; (2) there is such a prevalent lack of knowledge about services among the aged; (3) lack of knowledge is most prevalent among those at whom services are most directly aimed; (4) lack of information and sophistication is something we might be able to do something about.

There are at least three steps that I can see which would improve service delivery to aged.

First, education of those who are most out of touch with what is going on seems essential. I realize the practical problems in effecting education, and I'll blatantly duck the difficult issue of how to do it. However, for the foreseeable future, I suspect that our social services will continue to rely heavily on self-diagnosis. Therefore, if services are to be distributed in something at all comparable to the actual distribution of objective need, we have to make the most needy able to recognize needs for service when they have them.

Second, the level of information is sufficiently low that even the better informed will be vague about where they should go for service. There should probably be an easily accessible place for aged to call or visit where they can get quick and accurate information about whether or not a service exists that is appropriate for their problem. It has been well demonstrated that people who are vague about what they need will not persevere very long to get something. We need to make it easy. The system should not depend on the person getting to exactly the right agency with exactly the right description of his problem to make him look eligible. This, again, works against the people who are most needy but least informed.

Third, the whole concept of "outreach" is essentially getting away from placing the burden for diagnosis on the person himself. I gather this concept is being utilized in varying degrees in various settings. In addition, however, there are some professionals who have regular contact with aged who could help them assess their problems and could be funds of information about services available. Some aged have no contacts with such groups as Golden Age Clubs, which often serve this function. We know, however, that three-quarters of the aged see some doctor at least once a year. Perhaps doctors could help more. Perhaps there are other contacts which could also be utilized in this way, if the contacts themselves could be sensitized to the problem of lack of information.

Finally, there is a rather clear and important methodological implication of these data for those doing research on need for service. One cannot measure need for service by asking a person whether or not he needs it, or has ever needed it. We found very few of the poor, the less educated, or the very old who thought they had ever needed a service that they had not received. To use such a measure to assess a service system will surely generate support for the adequacy of the system for exactly the same reason that the present system does not work well now: the needy do not know what they need.

Age and the Utilization of Medical Aid in a Small Town

by DEREK L. PHILLIPS

IN RECENT YEARS there has been an increasing awareness that there are many sick people who never seek medical assistance and who are, officially at least, not classified as ill.[1] Several investigations have attempted to determine the number of persons manifesting symptoms of illness who never come to the attention of medical experts.

One of the earliest of these studies was the Peckham experiment in which 91 per cent of a preselected sample of individuals classified as healthy were diagnosed as having physiological defects or aberrations, while among those who felt sick, 60 per cent were not receiving care.[2] Breslow, reporting on the California Health Survey, noted that "a substantial amount of illness does not come to the attention of physicians. For example, about one-fifth of the rheumatism, one-fourth of the deafness, and almost one-third of the asthma and hay fever reported in the survey were not medically attended."[3] Koos in his study of "Regionville" found that

1. This research was conducted by Derek L. Phillips and Bernard E. Segal. It was supported by Grants CHOO82 and CHOO286 from the Division of Community Health Services, United States Public Health Service.
2. I. H. Pearse and L. H. Crocker, *The Peckham Experiment: A Study in the Living Structure of Society* (London: George Allen & Unwin, Ltd., 1961).
3. L. Breslow, "Uses and Limitations of the California Health Survey for Studying the Epidemiology of Chronic Disease," *American Journal of Public Health* 47 (1957): 168–73.

almost 25 per cent of the illnesses were not treated by a physician.[4] A more recent study of multiphasic screenings with almost 11,000 apparently healthy persons showed that 92 per cent had some disease or clinical disorder.[5] Similarly in England, a survey indicated that, despite the availability of free medical care, 37 per cent of the families studied had a member suffering pain or discomfort who was not seeking medical help.[6] These studies seem to reveal two important conclusions. First, there are many persons who, upon medical examination, turn out to have one or more medical disorders or illnesses—unbeknownst to themselves. And, second, there are a large number of individuals who define themselves as ill but do not seek medical assistance. The concern in the present paper is with this second group of individuals.

Before proceeding further with consideration of this study of illness and the utilization of medical help, it is necessary to say a few words about the use of the term illness. As Mechanic has noted, the term is frequently used in two ways by analysts who are concerned with issues of health and illness: "On the one hand, it refers to a limited scientific concept . . . and, on the other, to any condition which causes, or might usefully cause, an individual to concern himself with his symptoms and to seek help. The term 'illness behavior' refers to any behavior relevant to the second, more general, interpretation. If we are to understand the process of illness, it becomes necessary to consider what goes on even before a person sees a doctor or some other health worker. Thus the study of the patient's perspective is an indispensable aspect of the analysis of health and disease."[7]

It seems obvious, then, that the study of illness behavior requires study not only of those who seek care, but also of those who do not. Investigations of sick persons who do not seek help is especially important in that as many as two-thirds of those who re-

---

4. E. L. Koos, *The Health of Regionville* (New York: Columbia University Press, 1954).

5. J. E. Schenthal, "Multiphastic Screening of the Well Patient," *Journal of the American Medical Association* 172 (1960): 1–4.

6. Political and Economic Planning, *Family Needs and Social Services* (London: George Allen &: Unwin, Ltd., 1961).

7. David Mechanic, *Medical Sociology* (New York: Free Press, 1968), p. 115.

port illness in household interviews have been found not to seek a physician's advice.[8]

Most studies of the utilization of medical care have emphasized either economic or social–psychological factors as paramount in people's decisions to seek or not seek care. We have chosen to focus on the social–psychological factors, in that there is good reason to believe that they are of most importance in the community chosen for study. The present paper is one of a series of reports on the illness behavior of a sample of residents living in a small New England town.[9] These reports are concerned with the relationships of the recognition, definition, impact, and course of illness to a variety of social and social–psychological factors. Starting with the facts that not all ill people seek medical help, and that, of those who do, not all are equally likely to follow medical advice, this project set out to determine why laymen often think of illness and its treatment in terms different from physicians. The project also considers social factors which may keep laymen from dealing with their illnesses in what physicians would consider medically appropriate ways and then focuses on the question of what these differences between medical and lay views mean to the course of illness and resultant social disability. Patients, of course, play an active part in selecting their own alternative methods of dealing with illness. Social and social–psychological factors, therefore, come into play, affecting the decisions ill persons make regarding illness and responses to medical personnel. As Zola has noted, "It is not merely that there are social and psychological factors in illness but that illness is a social and psychological phenomenon. It cannot be understood or have any meaning without reference to a social context."[10]

This paper is concerned specifically with the relationship between people's ages and their help-seeking experiences when ill.

8. K. L. White *et al.*, "The Ecology of Medical Care," *New England Journal of Medicine* 265 (1961): 885–92.

9. The first of this series was Derek L. Phillips and Bernard E. Segal, "Sexual Status and Psychiatric Symptoms," *American Sociological Review* 34 (1969): 58–72.

10. Irving K. Zola, "Problems for Research—Some Effects of Assumptions Underlying Sociomedical Investigations," in G. Gordon (ed.), *Proceedings, Conference on Medical Sociology and Disease Control* (University of Chicago Center for Health Administration Studies, 1964), p. 17.

A further concern is with those sociocultural factors that may help to account for age differences in help-seeking behavior. What is attempted is to link age to social group structure and both of these to help-seeking behavior by means of an intervening set of medical orientation factors indicative of a scientific or popular approach to health and medical care.

METHODS

The study was carried out in Lebanon, New Hampshire, a small New England town of approximately 9,000 inhabitants. Respondents were selected randomly from the City Directory (1964), with the stipulation that the sample include only married persons between the ages of twenty-one and fifty. This stipulation hopefully means that differences in utilization will not be due to economic problems and serious illnesses associated with old age. An additional stipulation was that in no case should a husband and wife both be included in the sample. Our initial sample of 302 respondents (153 women and 149 men) was interviewed during the winter and spring of 1964–65. One year later, each of the sample members was contacted for a second interview. In the second wave of interviews, 278 of the original sample (141 women and 137 men) were reinterviewed. Thus, the sample "mortality" was only 8 per cent over the one-year period. The findings presented in this paper are based on the 278 respondents for whom we have data from two interviews spaced one year apart.

In addition to gathering data from respondents, we obtained data from the records of private physicians and from clinic and hospital records. Because of the small size of Lebanon and the fact that adjacent communities are smaller still, we were able to secure the cooperation of all health personnel with whom Lebanon residents might come into contact. Clearance was secured from the respondents for investigating their case records in physicians' offices, in the small local hospital in Lebanon and at Mary Hitchcock Hospital and Clinic in Hanover—the only major medical center within a radius of over fifty miles. The records of all physicians within the locality—there are no private physicians in Hanover— and the records of the hospitals and clinics were searched to determine each respondent's use of the medical services and facilities during the twelve-month period between the first and second interviews. We feel confident that we have managed to learn about almost all medical visits made by the people in our sample. Even those few patients who went outside the area for medical assistance did so after consulting with a local doctor or a physician at one of the local hospitals. Although our sample was drawn in such a way as to purposely exclude older persons, there was considerable range in the ages of our respondents. For purposes of analysis, therefore, they are divided into three age groups: under age thirty-five, thirty-five to forty-four, and forty-five years of age and over.

In the remainder of this paper, the mode of presentation is as follows: First, we consider the relationship between age and several factors thought to be important in determining whether or not ill persons seek medical assistance for their troubles. This is done with data collected during the first interview. Second, we examine differences in help-seeking patterns for those who were ill during the period between the first and second interviews. Finally, we investigate the extent to which age differences in help-seeking during the second year of the study are accounted for by measures obtained in the first interview.

FINDINGS

Taking our cue from the work of Edward Suchman,[11] we first examined the relationship between age and an index of social organization. He labeled this dimension as "cosmopolitanism–parochialism," with the cosmopolitan end of the index indicative of heterogeneous and loosely knit interpersonal relationships and the parochial end indicative of homogeneous and closely knit interpersonal relationships. In the words of Suchman: "This measure may be taken to indicate the degree of identification of an individual with a parochial or limited, traditional, narrowly confined and closely knit 'in-group' point of view, as opposed to a cosmopolitan or more worldly, progressive, 'urban' or less personal way of life."[12]

11. "Sociomedical Variations Among Ethnic Groups," *American Journal of Sociology* 70 (1964): 319–31.
12. Suchman, p. 325.

Health Care Services for the Aged

The index of social organization employed in this research is similar to Suchman's and is based on responses to four questions: (1) Are most of your friends of the same nationality as you are? (2) Are most of your friends of the same religion as you are? (3) Are most of your friends people you grew up with? and (4) Are most of your close friends also friends with each other? In every case, a positive answer was scored as a parochial response and the scores ran from 0 (the cosmopolitan end of the scale) through 4 (the parochial end). In this report, those with scores of 0 and 1 are classified as cosmopolitans and those with scores of 2–4 are categorized as parochials.

TABLE 1

RELATIONSHIP BETWEEN AGE AND TYPE OF
SOCIAL ORGANIZATION

TYPE OF SOCIAL ORGANIZATION	AGE		
	Under 35 (N=91)	35–44 (N=116)	45+ (N=71)
Cosmopolitan	50.5%	50.0%	35.2%
Parochial	49.5%	50.0%	64.8%

Table 1 presents the relationship between age and people's classification on the index of social organization. Inspection of this table reveals that the percentage of parochials increases as we look across the table from left to right. Whereas fewer than one-half of the respondents under age thirty-five are parochials, almost two-thirds of those in the age group forty-five and over are classified as parochials. A similar pattern was found for each of the four items in the index. Since we were also interested in establishing the stability of the relationship between age and type of social organization, it was examined under separate controls for sex and social class position. Under each of the controls, the relation between age and type of social organization was maintained.

Like Suchman, we felt that "the more ethnocentric and cohesive the social group, the more isolated and alienated it will be from the larger society and the less likely it will be to accept the objectives and methods of the formal medical care system."[13] More specifi-

13. Suchman, p. 323.

94

cally, it was expected that older persons, especially if they were parochials, would be less likely than younger ones to engage in preventive medical behavior and would be more apt than others to have negative attitudes toward medical care. For *preventive medical behavior,* one simple indicator was used. That was responses to the question: Do you get periodical medical checkups when you are not ill? Attitudes toward medical care were estimated by two indexes, each consisting of two items. The index of *skepticism* toward medical care had two items: (1) Have you ever had any questions or skeptical thoughts about the way a doctor handled your case? and (2) I have my doubts about some things doctors say they can do for you, with a "yes" answer to the first question and an "agree" answer to the second indicating skepticism. *Physician's interest* in patients' welfare was measured by responses to the questions: (1) As compared to the prices you have to pay for other things these days, do you think that doctors' charges are: a bargain, just about right, too much? and (2) Most doctors are more interested in their patients' welfare than anything else. Answers of too much and disagree were scored as indicating a negative attitude toward physicians' interest.

Table 2 allows for examination of both the independent and joint effects of age and type of social organization on preventive medical behavior, skepticism, and view of physician's interest. Looking at the top third of the table, we can see the following with regard to preventive medical behavior: (1) for both parochials and cosmopolitans, older persons are less likely than younger ones to seek medical checkups; (2) in each age group, parochials are less likely than cosmopolitans to engage in preventive medical behavior; and (3) strong joint effects on seeking checkups are exercised by age and type of social organization. At one extreme, among persons under age thirty-five who have a cosmopolitan orientation, only 24.9 per cent of the respondents report that they do not seek preventive medical care; at the other, among those over age forty-five who are parochials, almost 60 per cent fail to obtain medical checkups when they are not ill.

Looking at the relationships of the other two measures to age and type of social organization, the patterns are much less clear. Neither skepticism nor physician's interest bears any consistent

relationship to age. With regard to their relation to social organization, there is a slight tendency for attitudes to be more negative
among parochials. This is the case in the youngest and oldest
groups, although not among those thirty-five to forty-four. Later
we will explore the extent to which these three factors relate to the
actual *behavior* of people who become ill.

We now come to our examination of age differences in the utilization of medical aid among those who were ill during the period

TABLE 2

RELATIONSHIP BETWEEN AGE, TYPE OF SOCIAL ORGANIZATION,
AND HEALTH-RELATED INDEXES

HEALTH-RELATED INDEXES	AGE					
	Under 35		35–44		45+	
	Cosmo. (N=46)	Paroch. (N=45)	Cosmo. (N=58)	Paroch. (N=58)	Cosmo. (N=25)	Paroch. (N=46)
Preventive Medical Behavior						
Low Score	24.9%	35.6%	29.3%	44.8%	44.0%	58.7%
Skepticism of Medical Care						
High Score	37.0%	44.5%	45.5%	37.9%	24.0%	43.5%
Physician's Interest in Patients' Welfare						
Low interest	32.6%	44.4%	44.8%	37.6%	20.0%	32.6%

between the two interviews. The presence of illness was measured
in the following manner. People were asked whether or not they
had a number of specific illnesses or physical difficulties. A standard
medical checklist was utilized, and people were asked about such
things as bronchitis, ulcers, diabetes, asthma, and so forth. Our
original intention was to match people with the identical illnesses
and then observe differences in the seeking of medical help. The
limitations of this will be discussed later. The checklist contained
some thirty-one items, although for nine of them (pneumonia, T.B.,
diabetes, nervous breakdown, fainting, twitching, stammering or
stuttering, frigidity, and disturbed potency) none of the respondents reported that they had had any of them "in the year or so

since you were last interviewed." For fourteen of these items the oldest age group had the highest percentage reporting such troubles, and for eight there were virtually no differences in the various age groups. It is not surprising, of course, that older persons should be in poorer health than younger ones.

With regard to whether people were ill at all, there were almost no differences among the three age groups. This is somewhat unexpected, as one would anticipate fewer "illness-free" persons among those forty-five and over than in the other two age groups. Among those who were ill, however, those in the oldest age group were most likely to have a large number of illnesses; 16.4 per cent of those under age thirty-five, 17.2 per cent of those between thirty-five and forty-four, and 22.5 per cent of those forty-five and over reported five or more illnesses or physical difficulties.

As was noted earlier, the original intention was to match people of different ages with various physical illnesses and then to compare their help-seeking behavior. This turned out not to be possible because of the small sample size, the great variety of physical illnesses reported, and the rather small percentage of respondents reporting any given illness. Therefore, we turn our attention to the relationship between age and seeking medical aid among those who were *ill at all* during the period between the two interviews. The utilization of medical aid was determined by a thorough check of physicians' records and of the records contained in the small local hospital in Lebanon and at Mary Hitchcock Hospital and Clinic in Hanover.

Since those in the oldest age group have the largest number of illnesses, we might expect our analysis to show a higher rate of help-seeking in this group than among younger respondents. However, looking at Table 3 we can see that this is not the case. Despite the fact that they have a larger number of illnesses, they have the smallest percentage of persons who sought medical help. Whereas almost 80 per cent of those under age thirty-five have obtained medical assistance when ill, 68.1 per cent of those 35 to 44, and 61.5 per cent of the respondents over age forty-five sought medical aid— a difference between the youngest and oldest groups of about 18 percentage points.

In the next table we look at the help-seeking patterns of those who *did seek help.* For purposes of presentation here, they are divided into three categories: (1) those visiting a private physician only; (2) those visiting a private physician plus a clinic and/or hospital; and (3) those visiting a clinic and/or hospital, but not a private physician. Examination of Table 4 reveals that in all three age

TABLE 3

RELATIONSHIP BETWEEN AGE AND HELP-SEEKING
(*Among Ill Persons*)

Help-Seeking Behavior	Age		
	Under 35 (N=83)	35–44 (N=108)	45+ (N=65)
Not Seeking Help	20.5%	31.9%	38.5%
Seeking Help	79.5%	68.1%	61.5%

groups, consultation solely with a private physician is the most common experience, although the figure for those over age forty-five is much lower than for the other persons. The oldest group, however, has the highest percentage of individuals who have sought help directly from a clinic and/or hospital without first seeing a private physician. More than 30 per cent of those in the oldest age group have this pattern as compared to about 15 per cent in the other two groups.

TABLE 4

HELP-SEEKING PATTERNS OF ILL PERSONS

Pattern of Help	Age		
	Under 35 (N=66)	35–44 (N=71)	45+ (N=39)
Private physician only	59.1%	60.6%	41.0%
Private physician plus clinic and/or hospital	24.2%	25.3%	28.2%
Clinic and/or hospital, but not private physician	16.7%	14.1%	30.8%

We now turn to an exploration of whether or not the relationship between age and help-seeking is in any way due to the fact that younger persons are more apt to be cosmopolitans and older ones parochials, and that it is this rather than age *per se* that affects help-seeking. If this is the case, then the percentage point difference between the younger and older respondents observed in Table 3 should be reduced when people are classified by type of social organization. Looking at Table 5, we see that this is only partially true. Among respondents with a cosmopolitan orientation, the difference between the youngest and oldest age groups is reduced to 13 percentage points. However, the percentage point difference among parochials is 22 percentage points, a somewhat larger difference than was seen in Table 3. Furthermore, it is clear that age has a greater influence than type of social organization on whether or not people seek medical assistance for their illnesses. Also worth

TABLE 5

HELP-SEEKING BY AGE AND TYPE OF SOCIAL ORGANIZATION
(Percentage Not Seeking Help)

SOCIAL ORGANIZATION	AGE		
	Under 35	35–44	45+
Cosmopolitans	16.3%	29.6%	29.2%
	(N=43)	(N=54)	(N=24)
Parochials	25.0%	35.6%	48.8%
	(N=40)	(N=54)	(N=41)

stressing is the strong joint influence of age and type of social organization on help-seeking. Only 16.3 per cent of the young cosmopolitan respondents failed to seek medical help as compared to almost 50 per cent of the older parochial respondents.

Let us now see whether type of social organization has any effects on the relationship between age and *where* people seek help. Examining Table 6 we see that the patterns found in Table 4 hold true for both parochials and cosmopolitans; older respondents are less likely than younger ones to go directly to a clinic and/or hospital without first seeing a private physician. There are also, however, differences between parochials and cosmopolitans. Within all three age groups, a higher percentage of parochials than cosmopolitans utilize a private physician together with a clinic and or hospital. And within each age group, a higher percentage of cosmopolitans than parochials use a clinic and/or hospital but not a private physician. Clearly, then, both age and type of social organization exercise an influence on the help-seeking patterns of ill persons who do choose to seek medical assistance. Perhaps the most notable demonstration of the *joint* effects of these two factors on where people go for help is the fact that among young persons with a parochial orientation, 63.3 per cent see only a private physician and 10.0 per cent utilize a clinic and/or hospital; whereas among cosmopolitans over the age of forty-five, 35.3 per cent see only a private physician and 47.0 per cent utilize a clinic and/or hospital.

TABLE 6

HELP-SEEKING PATTERNS OF ILL PERSONS BY AGE AND TYPE OF
SOCIAL ORGANIZATION

PATTERN OF HELP	AGE					
	Under 35		35–44		45+	
	Cosmo. (N=36)	Paroch. (N=30)	Cosmo. (N=38)	Paroch. (N=33)	Cosmo. (N=17)	Paroch. (N=22)
Private physician only	55.6%	63.3%	65.8%	54.5%	35.3%	45.5%
Private physician plus clinic and/or hospital	22.3%	26.7%	15.8%	33.3%	17.7%	36.3%
Clinic and/or hospital, but not private physician	22.1%	10.0%	18.4%	12.2%	47.0%	18.2%

We now return to a further consideration of *why* ill persons do not seek medical assistance when they are ill. We have already seen that older persons are less likely to seek medical aid than younger ones and that this is especially the case when we compare young cosmopolitans with older parochials. It should be recalled that we saw in an earlier table (Table 2) that whether or not people get a medical checkup is dependent on both their age and their type of social organization. Let us now consider whether those who get such checkups differ from those who do not in regard to seeking medical help. We will consider this possibility by examining the relationship under a simultaneous control for age and type of social organization.

Table 7 allows for examination of all three factors—age, type of organization, and preventive medical care—as they influence help-seeking among ill persons. In that the resulting patterns are somewhat complex, they demand rather extensive discussion. The first thing to be observed is that people who do seek preventive health care are more likely than persons not seeking such health care to have sought help if they are ill. That is, people who regularly get checkups are more likely than others to seek medical assistance when ill. This is true in all three age groups and for both parochials and cosmopolitans. Apparently, then, taking the precautions suggested by the medical profession is part of a more "scien-

TABLE 7

HELP-SEEKING BY AGE, TYPE OF SOCIAL ORGANIZATION, AND
PREVENTIVE MEDICAL BEHAVIOR
(*Percentage not seeking help*)

Preventive Medical Behavior	Age					
	Under 35		35–44		45+	
	Cosmo.	Paroch.	Cosmo.	Paroch.	Cosmo.	Paroch.
Checkups	15.2%	24.0%	25.6%	30.0%	21.4%	29.4%
	(N=33)	(N=25)	(N=39)	(N=30)	(N=14)	(N=17)
No Checkups	20.0%	26.7%	40.0%	50.0%	40.0%	54.2%
	(N=10)	(N=15)	(N=15)	(N=24)	(N=10)	(N=24)

tific" orientation that is associated with help-seeking behavior when ill. More will be said shortly about this scientific orientation.

Let us now try to unravel the rather complex relationship involving these different influences on medical help-seeking. Looking at the relationship between age and help-seeking, we find something rather interesting. Among people who obtain checkups, the relation between age and help-seeking is much weaker than was originally seen in Table 3. Comparing the youngest and oldest age groups, there is a difference of about 6 percentage points among cosmopolitans and 5 percentage points among parochials. Among those who do not seek checkups, however, the age group differences are larger than originally seen: 20 percentage points among cosmopolitans and approximately 27 points among those with a parochial orientation. In other words, the independent effects of age are considerably more pronounced among people who fail to seek preventive medical care than among those who do so.

Examining the independent effects of type of social organization on help-seeking, we see no clear pattern as regards whether type of social organization is more pronounced among parochials or cosmopolitans, although in every comparison, type of social organization does make a difference in whether or not people seek help.

Looking at the independent effects of preventive medical behavior on help-seeking, we see another pattern in Table 7. Among respondents under age thirty-five, whether or not people regularly get checkups has virtually no effect on their subsequent illness behavior. Among those persons in the other two groups, however, preventive medical care makes a sizeable difference. For those thirty-five to forty-four, it makes a difference of 14 percentage points for cosmopolitans and 20 points for parochials. And for people forty-five and older, preventive medical practice makes a difference of 19 percentage points among cosmopolitans and 25 percentage points among parochials.

Considering the individual effects of each of the three factors on help-seeking, age and preventive medical care exercise about the same degree of influence, with type of social organization having considerably less effect. And, of course, it is worth emphasizing the strong joint effects of the three factors on people's illness behavior. At the one extreme where we have younger cosmopolitans who seek regular checkups, only 15.2 per cent did not seek medical help when ill; while at the other extreme, where we have parochials over age forty-five who do not seek regular checkups, 54.2 per cent did not seek medical assistance.

In the following two tables, the mode of analysis is similar to what was seen in Table 7. However, it differs in one important respect. Whereas in Table 7 preventive medical care was seen as a variable that might help account for the previously demonstrated relationship involving age, type of social organization, and help-seeking, skepticism and view of physician's interest are not to be considered in the same way. That is, since preventive medical care was related to age and type of social organization, it was appropriate to consider it as a variable that might intervene between these variables and help-seeking. However, skepticism and view of physician's interest, as we saw in Table 2, bear no consistent relation to age and type of social organization.

Turning now to Table 8, we have the introduction of "skepticism of medical care" into the analysis. We see that people who have a skeptical attitude about medical care are less likely to seek help when ill than are people who are not skeptical. This is true in all age groups and for both parochials and cosmopolitans. Whether or not people are skeptical does, then, have an influence on their illness behavior. Once again, age and type of social organization continue to exert an independent influence on help-seeking behavior. And the three variables considered together exercise a

TABLE 8

HELP-SEEKING BY AGE, TYPE OF SOCIAL ORGANIZATION, AND PHYSICIAN SKEPTICISM
(Percentage not seeking help)

Skepticism	Age					
	Under 35		35–44		45+	
	Cosmo.	Paroch.	Cosmo.	Paroch.	Cosmo.	Paroch.
High	20.0%	29.4%	33.3%	50.0%	40.0%	50.0%
	(N=15)	(N=17)	(N=27)	(N=22)	(N= 5)	(N=18)
Low	14.2%	21.7%	25.9%	31.2%	26.3%	39.1%
	(N=28)	(N=23)	(N=27)	(N=32)	(N=19)	(N=23)

strong cumulative influence. Approximately 14 per cent of the young cosmopolitans who have a positive attitude toward medical care fail to seek help when ill, while 50 per cent of the older parochials with a skeptical attitude toward medical care fail to seek medical assistance.

Table 9 examines the second index of attitude toward medical care, "physician's interest in patients' welfare," as it relates to illness behavior. Although the independent influence of this variable on help-seeking is rather modest among parochials and cosmopolitans alike in the two younger age groups, it quite markedly affects those over age forty-five. Age and type of social organization continue to show an independent influence and the three variables work together to influence help-seeking. Fewer than 14 per cent of the young cosmopolitans who see physicians as having a high interest in their welfare fail to obtain medical help, as compared with 61.5 per cent of the oldest parochials who see physicians as having low interest in their welfare.

Taking all of these findings together, we can create composite pictures of two types of individuals with regard to illness behavior. These are, of course, ideal types, although a few of our respondents do show all of the characteristics to be mentioned for each type. Despite this fact, it is useful to discuss these two ideal types in somewhat greater detail. For purposes of further discussion we shall refer to these two types simply as "seekers" and "non-seekers." Non-seekers are people over age forty-five, whose friends are people they grew up with, whose friends are of the same religion and nationality, and whose friends are friends of one another. From

TABLE 9

HELP-SEEKING BY AGE, TYPE OF SOCIAL ORGANIZATION, AND
VIEW OF PHYSICIANS' INTEREST
(*Percentage not seeking help*)

View of Physicians' Interest	Age					
	Under 35		35–44		45+	
	Cosmo.	Paroch.	Cosmo.	Paroch.	Cosmo.	Paroch.
Low	21.4%	26.9%	30.4%	40.0%	40.0%	61.5%
	(N=14)	(N=19)	(N=23)	(N=15)	(N= 5)	(N=13)
High	13.8%	23.8%	29.0%	38.5%	26.8%	35.7%
	(N=29)	(N=21)	(N=31)	(N=39)	(N=19)	(N=28)

what we know of other studies of cosmopolitans and parochials (usually referred to as locals),[14] they are probably more oriented to what happens in their home community than what happens elsewhere. They are narrow in their outlook, with their horizons seldom extending beyond the town where they live. This narrowness of horizon seems to be reflected in a popular health orientation, with an emphasis on a subjective, informal, lay, dependent, orientation to health and health services.[15] This is evidenced by a lack of concern with preventive medical practices and generally negative attitudes toward medical care.

The other type, the seekers, are people of less than thirty-five years of age, whose friends are likely to be of different ethnic and religious backgrounds, and whose friends are likely to be people

14. See, for example, Alvin W. Gouldner, "Cosmopolitans and Locals: Toward an Analysis of Latent Social Roles—I," *Administrative Science Quarterly* 2 (1957): 281–306.
15. Suchman.

they met as adults rather than people they grew up with. They are probably oriented to national issues, to matters outside the community where they reside. Their broadness of interest is evidenced in a scientific health orientation, emphasizing an objective, formal, professional, independent approach to health matters.[16] These individuals generally engage in preventive medical practices and have favorable attitudes toward medical care and the health professions.

In discussing the relationship between age and the utilization of health services by ill people, primary emphasis in this report has been placed on the social structural and social psychological factors that intervene between age and utilization. This is not to deny that economic factors may also play a part in determining whether or not people seek help for their medical problems. However, it was found in our analysis of the data collected during the first year's interviews that very few persons mentioned economic considerations as important factors in their illness behavior. For instance, in response to the question, "Would you, yourself, go to the doctor more often if it were not for the expense involved?" fewer than 8 per cent of the respondents said that this was definitely the case for them. This may be due partially to the fact that more than 90 per cent of those in the study said that they had health insurance. Another indicator of the general unimportance of economic considerations in regard to the utilization of medical services is the finding that only 15 per cent of the respondents reported that their "last medical expense" caused them *any* financial problems.

Thus while medical expenses are a source of great concern to the vast majority of Americans, the residents of Lebanon, New Hampshire do not seem to view financial considerations as particularly crucial in determining their illness behavior. This is probably due to a combination of factors: the fact that there is very little unemployment in the area, that the vast majority of people have health insurance, and that both local physicians in Lebanon and the surrounding area and the Mary Hitchcock Hospital and Clinic in Hanover are willing to forego immediate payment from patients without adequate financial resources.

While Lebanon, New Hampshire, is obviously in no way a repre-

16. Suchman.

sentative community, it is our view that the relationships shown to operate there are likely to be found in other communities and health-settings as well. Hopefully, the findings set forth in this report point to some of the myriad of factors that account for the unwillingness of many ill people to seek medical help.

Standards for the Audit and Planning of Medical Care: With Illustrations from Myocardial Infarction

by HYMAN K. SCHONFELD

THERE ARE many factors that govern the utilization of health services. Some factors are more relevant today, while others undoubtedly will exert greater influence in the future. Many of these factors, moreover, have a differential effect so that all categories of persons are not affected similarly.

Professionally defined health needs are describable in part by incidence, prevalence, recurrent attack, cure, and death rates. The magnitudes of these rates are dependent upon how professionals classify diseases, when they believe that professional assistance is required, what kinds of services should be provided, and when they think that such services are no longer necessary. Much of the preceding, of course, is dependent upon prior actions of individuals for practitioners often cannot do anything—except for certain community wide measures—unless the individual is available for services. Moreover, practitioners usually cannot identify needs for individuals unless these persons contact them. Therefore, fundamental to this professional concept of need is the individual's prior and continuing action in the form of demand.

Stated simply, demand follows a progression from the person's *recognition* that something is wrong, to the feeling that care of some type should be sought, to the *motivation* to actually seek such care.

Health Care Services for the Aged

Depending upon the ability of the motivated individual to actively seek care, an ability partly determined by the person's financial and physical conditions, this progression may be finally culminated as an *effective demand,* i.e., the person has care provided to him. As can be imagined, an individual often does not have complete control over what occurs at each step in this chain of events. A variety of societal influences are among the factors that shape the picture of needs and demands at any given time. These factors range widely and include such items as: (1) Legislation concerning the financing and provision of health care—whether this legislation is for selected groups in governmental programs (e.g., Medicare or Medicaid) or for those having other types of health insurance; the latter influencing the actions of Blue Cross Associations, Blue Shield Associations, commercial insurance carriers, or sponsors of private health plans. (2) Professionally related activities of health practitioners whether as individuals or as members of organizations. (3) Educational and persuasive techniques, such as those conducted by pharmaceutical companies through their advertisements in mass communications media.

The above factors, as well as many others, influence—consciously or unconsciously—what actually occurs during the progression process from the recognition of the need for care to the receipt of care by individuals from health practitioners. Some of these factors may lead to overutilization of services, whereas other factors may result in underutilization. The concept of over- and underutilization implies that there is a predetermined acceptable level of utilization. Both over- and underutilization may result from the actions or lack of actions of either the patient, the professional or both. Because of the additional burden that overutilization places on the limited supply of health professionals and facilities, because overutilization may also unnecessarily increase expenditures, and because in some instances either over- or underutilization may adversely affect the person's health, it becomes increasingly important for people to *receive the amounts and kinds of care that should be given* to them rather than what they are presently receiving—if these two measures of care are not the same.

Several methods can be (and have been) used to determine the acceptable level of care that people *should* receive. Two of these

108

methods consider that the care that certain people now receive should be the care that all similar patients should receive. One of these two methods is based on the theory that the care that experts provide to their patients should be the kind of care that is best for all patients under similar circumstances. However, it is still possible that this care may represent over- or underutilization when compared to some predetermined set of standards. A second method, the "end result" method, is based on the assumption that the care received by individuals who have favorable outcomes is the kind of care that should be provided to all patients of this type. This method, however otherwise commendable, is subject to the disadvantages that for some diseases or conditions favorable outcomes may be difficult to describe and/or measure, or that long periods of time may be required before the outcomes can be evidenced. An assumption is made in this method that the favorable outcome is somehow associated with the care provided.

A third method used to determine the amounts and kinds of care that people should receive is based on the opinions of professionally respected practitioners as to what they think *should* be done for persons having one or another disease or condition. This method assumes that these knowledgeable practitioners will give opinions tempered by their own clinical experiences and their knowledge of the clinical literature, as well as by their professional judgments as to what should be done, thus perhaps providing standards that are more or less independent of those practices that currently may result in over- or underutilization. The Department of Epidemiology and Public Health, School of Medicine, Yale University, is presently employing this method.

YALE STUDIES ON STANDARDS FOR GOOD CARE

Physicians and dentists who are in private practice in the New Haven area, and who also hold appointments on the Clinical Faculty of the Yale School of Medicine, are asked to give their opinions as to what should be done for the prevention of specific diseases and for the diagnosis, treatment, and follow-up of persons with a particular disease or condition. The objectives of these studies include the development of indexes and standards that can be used to describe what should be done for individuals if good care is to be provided for them. These standards can also be used in the planning of health services, in the estimation of needed personnel and facilities, in the estimation of projected costs, in the education of health practitioners, and in the audit of care that has been provided to patients with one or another disease.

Initially, these studies are based on interviews with physicians, dentists, nurses, social workers, etc. concerning what they think should be done if people are to receive good care. To date, "primary-physician" internists have been interviewed on 170 adult diseases; primary-physician pediatricians on 81 diseases affecting children. The opinions obtained relate to the services that should be provided for a specific disease or condition having regard for the following.

The kinds of services and amounts of each, i.e., the number of visits, the kinds and numbers of diagnostic and follow-up tests and procedures, treatment procedures, appliances, consultations, etc. required for the diagnosis, treatment, and follow-up of individuals according to: (1) the *kind of practitioner* who should provide the service e.g., a primary-physician internist, a "primary-physician" pediatrician, or a referral specialist, such as a cardiologist, neurologist, surgeon, etc.; (2) the *location*—physician's office, patient's home, hospital bed, etc.—at which the service should be provided, and; (3) the *sequence* in which these services should occur.

These sequences can be considered from the viewpoint of: (a) attacks or flare-ups, i.e., the first attack, the second attack, etc.; (b) the phase of care, i.e., the diagnostic period, the first year of treatment and follow-up, or each additional year of treatment and follow-up; (c) professional attention, i.e., the first attendance (phone call or visit), the second attendance, etc.; or (d) the nature of the attention, i.e., for those patients having diagnosis only, treatment only, or diagnosis *and* treatment by a particular type of practitioner.

The time involved in providing this care. This time (i.e., the number of minutes or hours required) can be discussed with reference to: (1) each service separately or similar kinds of services grouped together; (2) each visit separately or all visits combined; (3) the diagnostic, treatment, or follow-up periods separately, or

110

all combined; or (4) each attack separately, or the entire disease or condition considered as one entity.

Following the collection of these kinds of data from the individual physicians or dentists, these data are edited, tabulated, and reviewed. For some diseases and conditions these preliminary data have been reviewed by other practitioners on an individual basis, whereas for other diseases these reviews have taken place at sessions at which many (up to ten) reviewers have been present. Where necessary, changes are made in the preliminary standards. It is important to emphasize that even these revised standards must not be considered as final or permanent as they must be reviewed periodically and altered as required by changing medical practices. Moreover, these standards, prepared in one limited geographic area and by practitioners in one mode of practice, may not apply elsewhere. We encourage practitioners in other geographic locations and in other forms of practice to review these standards and to modify them as they think necessary.

The data derived from the interviews with the practitioners have been analyzed and are being presented in a number of ways. These data can be utilized for various purposes. Some of the methods of analysis and presentation and some of the proposed applications have been discussed in other papers and were concerned mainly with: indexes and standards for a variety of items;[1] pathways among primary physicians and specialists;[2] the application of the standards in estimating needed personnel, given the details of a program, the standards of good care, and the incidence

1. I. S. Falk, H. K. Schonfeld, B. R. Harris, S. J. Landau, and S. S. Milles, "The Development of Standards for the Audit and Planning of Medical Care: 1. Concepts, Research Design, and the Content of Primary Physician's Care," *American Journal of Public Health* 57 (July, 1967): 1118–36. H. K. Schonfeld, I. S. Falk, H. R. Sleeper, and W. D. Johnston, "The Content of Good Dental Care: Methodology in a Formulation for Clinical Standards and Audits, and Preliminary Findings," *American Journal of Public Health* 57 (July, 1967): 1137–46. H. K. Schonfeld, I. S. Falk, H. R. Sleeper, and W. D. Johnston, "Professional Dental Standards for the Content of Dental Examinations," *Journal of the American Dental Association* 77 (October, 1968): 870–77.

2. H. K. Schonfeld, I. S. Falk, P. H. Lavietes, S. S. Milles, and S. J. Landau, "The Development of Standards for the Audit and Planning of Medical Care: Pathways Among Primary Physicians and Specialists for Diagnosis and Treatment," *Medical Care* 6 (March-April, 1968): 101–14.

and prevalence of a disease;[3] the audit of hospital outpatient care;[4] and standards for a mixture of "first year" and "carry-over" patients.[5]

PATHWAYS OF GOOD CARE

This paper, while utilizing many of the concepts and formulas described in previous publications, focuses on the preparation and presentation of pathways of good care for individuals who have had a specific disease or condition. By (a) applying the indexes and standards of good care (the professional-logistics) derived from the opinions of the interviewed physicians (b) to the pathways of disease experienced by patients who have had one or more attacks of a disease (c) descriptions of "pathways of good care" are produced. Estimates can be made of the number of each kind of service required, the time involved, and the personnel (manpower) and facilities needed for the pathways of care associated with that disease or condition by taking into account the proportions of persons involved at each stage along the pathways. It should be understood, moreover, that within each of these broad pathways there may be secondary pathways, such as those based on referrals between primary physicians and specialists.

The simplest set of overall pathways are required for individuals having an acute disease which usually has only one attack —such as a communicable disease which may produce immunity. Figure 1 illustrates the four major pathways within this set. The terminal state of each pathway is indicated by the number 1, 2, 3, or 4 in Figure 1.

Many more, and more complex, sets of pathways must be con-

3. H. K. Schonfeld, I. S. Falk, P. H. Lavietes, J. Landwirth, and L. S. Krassner, "The Development of Standards for the Audit and Planning of Medical Care: Good Pediatric Care—Program Content and Method of Estimating Needed Personnel," *American Journal of Public Health* 58 (November, 1968): 2097–2110.

4. H. K. Schonfeld, "The Development of Standards for the Audit and Planning of Medical Care: Audit of Hospital Outpatient Care," in *Outpatient Care Audit*, the proceedings of a conference sponsored by University Hospitals, University of Minnesota Health Sciences Center, Minneapolis, March, 1968.

5. H. K. Schonfeld, "Standards for the Audit and Planning of Medical Care: A Method for Preparing Audit Standards for Mixtures of Patients," *Medical Care* (in press, May–June, 1970, issue).

FIGURE 1

PATHWAYS FOR AN ACUTE DISEASE OR CONDITION—WITH NO REPEAT ATTACKS*

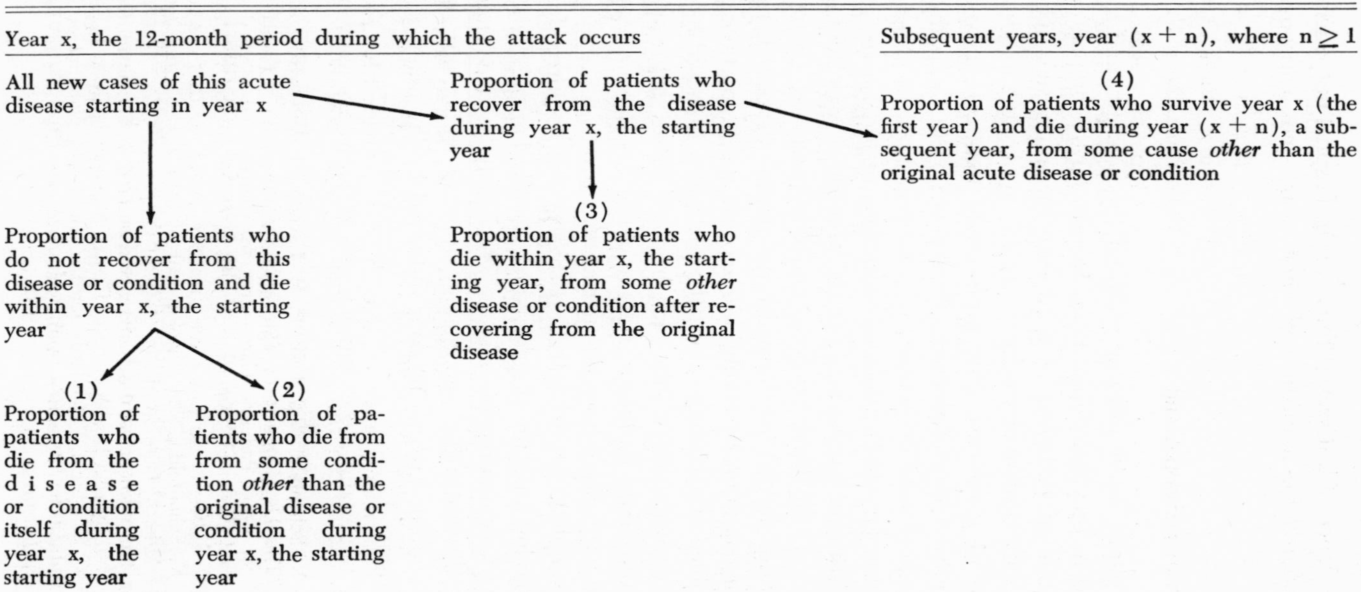

Year x, the 12-month period during which the attack occurs | **Subsequent years, year $(x + n)$, where $n \geq 1$**

All new cases of this acute disease starting in year x

Proportion of patients who recover from the disease during year x, the starting year

(3) Proportion of patients who die within year x, the starting year, from some *other* disease or condition after recovering from the original disease

Proportion of patients who do not recover from this disease or condition and die within year x, the starting year

(1) Proportion of patients who die from the d i s e a s e or condition itself during year x, the starting year

(2) Proportion of patients who die from some condition *other* than the original disease or condition during year x, the starting year

(4) Proportion of patients who survive year x (the first year) and die during year $(x + n)$, a subsequent year, from some cause *other* than the original acute disease or condition

*By definition the definitive care for the "acute attack" lasts less than 12 months. However, care in addition to that normally required for persons who have not had this disease or condition may be required during year x or during any or each subsequent year because of residual effects or complications that may have arisen as a result of the disease.

113

sidered when discussing an acute disease or condition which can have repeated attacks and when the timing of these repeated attacks—if they occur—can vary from almost immediately after the onset of the disease to many years after the first attack. A chronic disease that has repeated flare-ups will have the same pathways of disease as that of an acute–repeat attack-type of disease. In the case of an acute disease having the possibility of repeat attacks, there may or may not be the need for care between attacks. For the chronic disease with the potential of repeated flare-ups, there may be some degree of intermittent or continuous treatment or attention required between flare-ups. Even when no additional flare-up occurs there is often the need for either intermittent or continuous care after the disease or condition has been recognized. Figure 2 illustrates some of the many pathways that are associated with an acute disease which is subject to the possibility of repeated attacks or for a chronic disease, whether or not there are repeated flare-ups.

For each disease or condition of these types, the simplest set of pathways of care is required by those individuals who have only one attack or flare-up. Even within this set there may be several (four) alternative pathways, depending upon the terminal state reached. The terminal state of each pathway is indicated by a number, one to four as shown in Figure 2; and these four pathways for patients who have only one attack can be seen to be identical to the four pathways of the "one attack only" type of disease, as illustrated in Figure 1. Of these four pathways, the two that are most *unfavorable* are followed by patients who die *during* their first attack, i.e., those pathways ending in terminal states one and two. This does not mean, however, that the care provided for those patients—at least from the professional–logistic viewpoint—was not good. The *most desirable* pathways of the one attack only set (i.e., those pathways ending in terminal states three and four) are associated with the recovery of patients from this one attack. Thereafter, these patients do not have another attack of this disease and they have the same risks of developing other diseases, or of dying, as do persons who never had this disease. However, they may need additional care beyond the active phase of the attack because of some residual effect or complication that may arise during or following the attack.

It should be evident that as the number of repeat attacks increases, the number and complexity of the pathways of good care for a disease also increases. In order to keep Figure 2 from becoming too complex, however, only two attacks have been shown. Naturally, if the number of attacks exceeds two there would be more pathways and terminal states than now shown in Figure 2.

The problem in being able to (a) apply standards of good care to (b) pathways of disease in order to (c) produce pathways of good care, is not in the preparation of indexes and standards of good care but rather in obtaining information regarding pathways of disease. As described previously, we can and are developing standards for good care for first attacks and for subsequent attacks, and for the first year of care and for each of the subsequent years of care following an attack, i.e., "per stage of the pathway." We have also ascertained from the physicians interviewed their opinions as to how many patients, of those who have an attack, should be seen beyond twelve months following the start of the attack and for how many additional years care should be provided.

Where a disease can have *only one attack,* these data, together with published incidence, prevalence and mortality data, are sufficient to describe the care that should be associated with the four major pathways of that disease as illustrated in Figure 1. It is often not easy, however, to prepare descriptions of pathways of good care for those diseases or conditions for which patients may have more than one attack as illustrated in Figure 2. Here the problem is with the ability to obtain data as to the proportion of patients who have followed each pathway of that disease. The difficulty is in knowing how many patients have had only one attack, or two attacks, or three attacks, etc., and what the mortality rates and the number of years of survival are for each of those attack groups. It would seem that the lack of these kinds of information results from the absence of available data on *lifetime histories of groups of patients.* For some diseases and/or for some age groups, special longitudinal studies have been conducted thereby making it possible to obtain these kinds of data for each pathway. Moreover, such information is often more readily available for hospitalized patients than for patients treated solely in private offices. Undoubtedly, there must be much more of these kinds of data available than is

115

FIGURE 2

Pathways for an acute disease or condition—with repeat attacks—or for a chronic disease with the potential of repeated flare-ups.*

Year x, the 12-month period during which the 1st attack occurs

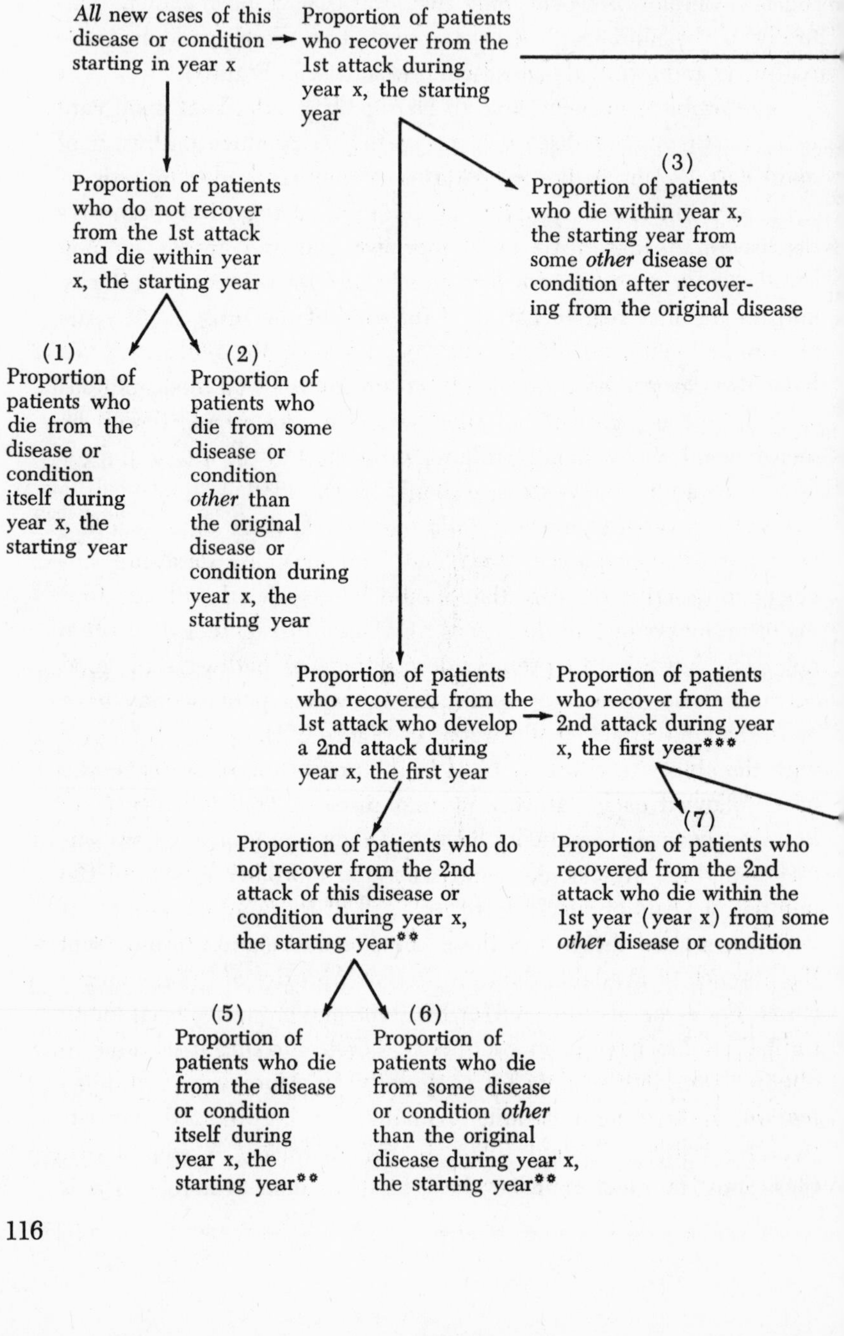

All new cases of this disease or condition starting in year x → Proportion of patients who recover from the 1st attack during year x, the starting year

Proportion of patients who do not recover from the 1st attack and die within year x, the starting year

(3) Proportion of patients who die within year x, the starting year from some *other* disease or condition after recovering from the original disease

(1) Proportion of patients who die from the disease or condition itself during year x, the starting year

(2) Proportion of patients who die from some disease or condition *other* than the original disease or condition during year x, the starting year

Proportion of patients who recovered from the 1st attack who develop a 2nd attack during year x, the first year

Proportion of patients who recover from the 2nd attack during year x, the first year***

Proportion of patients who do not recover from the 2nd attack of this disease or condition during year x, the starting year**

(7) Proportion of patients who recovered from the 2nd attack who die within the 1st year (year x) from some *other* disease or condition

(5) Proportion of patients who die from the disease or condition itself during year x, the starting year**

(6) Proportion of patients who die from some disease or condition *other* than the original disease during year x, the starting year**

Subsequent years, year $(x + n)$, where $n \geq 1$

roportion of patients who
ecover from the 1st attack
nd survive year x (the
rst year)

(4)
Proportion of patients who
recover from the first attack
and survive year x, the first
year, who die during a
subsequent year, year
$(x + n)$ from some cause
other than the original
disease or condition

roportion of patients who
ecovered from the 1st
ttack and survived year
the first year, who then
evelop another attack, a
nd attack, during a
ubsequent year, year
$(x + n)$

Proportion of patients who
recover from the 2nd attack,
the attack that occured
during the subsequent year,
year $(x + n)$***

(11)
Proportion of patients
who die within the
subsequent year, year
$(x + n)$ that the 2nd
attack occurred from
some cause *other* than
the original disease
or condition

roportion of patients who
ie from the 2nd attack,
hich occurred during the
ubsequent year, year
$(x + n)$****

(10)
Proportion of patients
having this 2nd attack
who die from some
disease or condition *other*
than the original
condition during the
subsequent year, year
$(x + n)$****

(9)
roportion of patients
aving this 2nd attack
ho die from the disease
condition itself
uring this subsequent
ear, year $(x + n)$****

(12)
Proportion of patients
who die within some
year subsequent to
the year $(x + n)$ in
which they recovered
from the 2nd attack,
from some cause
other than the original
disease or condition

(8)
Proportion of patients
who survived 2 attacks
during year x, who die
during a subsequent year,
year $(x + n)$ from some
cause *other* than the
original disease or condition

roportion of patients who
urvive the first year (year
) after recovering from
te second attack***

Note: this figure includes a maximum of only two attacks. The number of pathways would increase as the number of attacks increases beyond two.
  °By definition the definitive care for each "acute attack" lasts less than a 12
month period. However, care in addition to that normally required for persons who
have not had this disease or condition may be required during year x or during any
and each subsequent year because of residual effects or complications that may have
arisen as a result of the disease—regardless of which attack.
  °°Some patients die during year $(x + 1)$ as the second attack extends beyond 12
months from the beginning of the first attack.
  °°°Some patients may have a third attack or even more attacks.
  °°°°Some patients die during year $[x + (n + 1)]$ as the second attack may
extend beyond that year in which it occurs.

117

readily obtainable from published sources. However, it is necessary to have such data in order to be able to describe all the facets of all the pathways of care for a disease.

One factor that must be stressed in discussing pathways of disease, terminal states, and pathways of care is that at any given point in time the mixture of patients *alive* with a specific disease or condition consists of patients who will eventually be associated with one of the terminal states shown in Figures 1 or 2. Thus, the mixture of living patients is composed of a mixture of patients whose final outcome is still in doubt. At a point in time all that can be known about groups of living patients is how many have experienced (or are presently experiencing) specified stages of the disease pathway. That is, we can say how many patients have had one attack to date, or two attacks, etc., or how many patients have survived one attack (or two, or three) and are now in their first, or second, etc. year of treatment and/or follow-up, and so on. We can only classify *living* patients with regard to pathways of disease based on their experiences up to that point in time. As time progresses an individual may shift from one to another pathway group, depending upon the course of his disease experience. Knowledge about proportions of patients who have followed pathways that have led to each of the specified *terminal states* must be based on data obtained about patients who are no longer alive. We can use this knowledge to estimate the proportions of living patients who might be expected to follow each pathway if the present group of patients behave in the same manner as past patients. For obviously until the patient dies he cannot be positively identified with one or another terminal state and, therefore, with the unique pathway associated with that terminal state.

PATHWAYS OF GOOD CARE FOR MYOCARDIAL INFARCTION

The "lifetime" disease pathways for patients who have had myocardial infarcts follow closely all the pathways and terminal states shown in Figure 2. According to the physicians interviewed in the Yale study, the professional–logistic attention required of a physician for each attack of myocardial infarction should be relatively the same, that is, subsequent attacks should be diagnosed, treated and followed similar to first attacks. The number of visits per patient and the time per visit should be, on the average, the same for each attack—whether the first, second, third, etc.—except as variations are required to best meet the needs of individual patients. Moreover, these patients should have some degree of physician attention following an attack, or between attacks, and this attention should continue for the duration of the lifetime of the patient. This follow-up care, while not specifically for the treatment of the condition per se, allows the physician to keep an eye on the patient and to follow sequelae of the attack. It also serves a preventive function. The physician has the opportunity to determine whether the patient is following the recommended advice, possibly preventing recurrent attacks.

Table 1 gives data for each attack of myocardial infarction with respect to the attention required of a primary-physician internist by patients *who survive the attack.* Later, comments will be made about those patients who do not survive an attack. Although this table shows only average (mean) values, there is obviously a distribution of values as well as a range of values associated with each index and standard. Based on the opinions of the fifteen internists interviewed, the place of the first medical contact should be a hospital emergency room; though there is some feeling among these physicians that mobile cardiac units would be of considerable advantage to the patient as immediate attention could then be given at the site of the attack. The physicians indicated—though *not* shown in Table 1—that under present circumstances about 80 per cent of the patients should be seen initially in the emergency room with the other 20 per cent of the first contacts being equally divided between the physician's office and the patient's place of residence. Regardless of where this initial contact occurs, all patients should be hospitalized for treatment and in some of these cases for completion of the diagnosis.

Patients who survived an attack of myocardial infarction should have had, on the average, almost twenty-five hospital visits by primary-physician internists during the average of twenty-three days of hospitalization. The range for the number of these hospital visits may be between eighteen and thirty-seven, with 75 per cent or so of the patients requiring from twenty to twenty-four visits. The duration of the hospital stay may vary from two to over four weeks.

119

TABLE 1

Percentage of primary-physician internists' patients who survive an attack of myocardial infarction who should be seen by primary-physician internists for diagnosis, treatment, and follow-up, by location of visit, average number of visits per patient, and average time in minutes per visit per patient required during the attack and within a twelve month period following the start of the attack.

Location of attendance[a]	Diagnostic phase[b]			Treatment phase[b]			Diagnostic and treatment phases combined[b]		
	Percentage of patients[e]	Average number of visits per patient[e]	Average time per visit per patient[e]	Percentage of patients[e]	Average number of visits per patient[e]	Average time per visit per patient[e]	Percentage of patients[e]	Average number of visits per patient[e]	Average time per visit per patient[e]
			(minutes)			(minutes)			(minutes)
All locations[d]	100	1.5	28	100	30.1	22	100	31.6	23
Primary physician's office	11	1.1	30	100	4.5	30	100	4.6	30
Patient's home	11	1.1	37	80	2.0	30	80	2.2	31
Hospital emergency room	80	1.0	30	0	0	0	80	1.0	30
Hospital in-patient	16	2.8	23	100	24.0	20	100	24.5	20

Note: The data presented in this table are based on the opinions of the fifteen primary-physician internists interviewed in the Yale study. These data refer to the period of the attack and a twelve month period following the start of the attack.

a. A patient may be seen at more than one location for diagnosis and/or treatment.

b. These data apply to patients who survive the attack who should have been seen at the particular location indicated for the phase of care specified.

c. The percentage of patients, average number of visits per patient, and the average time per visit per patient refer to patients actually having visits with primary-physician internists at the specified location during the particular phase indicated.

d. The "all locations" data are *not* the sums of the data shown for the specific locations as a patient can be seen at more than one location. Also, the all locations data are based on values for each of the specified locations that were carried to more decimal places than those shown in this table.

During hospitalization the patients should undergo a number of diagnostic tests and procedures, as well as other tests to evaluate their conditions so that a proper course of therapy may be prescribed. Many of these tests are routine and definitely are not required solely for diagnostic purposes. During (and following) the period of hospitalization some of these same tests, as well as other tests and procedures, are indicated in order to periodically evaluate the patient's condition and progress. The tests and procedures recommended by the primary-physician internists and the percentages of surviving patients who should have these tests for diagnosis and/or treatment are shown in Table 2. As the number of times that a test should be performed are presented in this table as average values, it should be understood that some patients may require more whereas others may require fewer numbers of each test. For example, 50 per cent or so of the patients will probably require only one electrocardiogram in order to be able to say that a myocardial infarction had occurred; the remaining 50 per cent may require two, three or even more electrocardiograms in order to assist in establishing the diagnosis.

The treatment that the interviewed primary-physician internists thought necessary for patients who survived an attack of myocardial infarction is outlined in Table 3. What is not shown in this table are data on the use of coronary care units (ccu) and continuous monitoring. Extensive use of such units may necessitate changes in the professional–logistic data presented.

The interviewed internists thought that the need for consultation during the patient's stay in the hospital should be limited. Approximately 10 per cent of the patients (and mainly those with problems of arrhythmias) require consultations with cardiologists. Another 5 per cent or so of the patients, those who may require the insertion of either temporary or permanent pacemakers, should have consultations with vascular surgeons.

Interestingly enough, however, when six internist–cardiologists were interviewed concerning the care required for patients who had attacks of myocardial infarction, these cardiologists thought that approximately one-quarter of the primary-physician internists' patients should be referred to them. Referrals for approximately 4 per cent of the patients should be for diagnosis only, about 2 per cent for both diagnosis and treatment, and 17 per cent only for treatment. Table 4 gives visit and time data for those patients who should be referred to the cardiologist by the primary-physician internist and who survive the attack; and the percentages are given in terms of this group of patients as 100 per cent. It is interesting to

TABLE 2

Percentage of primary-physician internists' patients who survive an attack of myocardial infarction by kind and number of laboratory tests and other procedures required by primary-physician internists for establishing the diagnosis, evaluating the patients' condition, establishing a baseline for management and follow-up, and for managing and following the patient during the attack, and within a twelve-month period following the start of the attack.

Test or procedure	For diagnosis, evaluation and baseline		For management and follow-up[a]	
	Percentage of patients	Number of tests[b]	Percentage of patients	Number of tests[b]
Chest x-ray	100	1	100	2
Complete blood count	100	1	25	2.5
Electrocardiograph	100	2	100	10
Stool for blood	100[c]	1	15	12
Urinalysis	100	1	100	2.8
VDRL	100	1	0	0
Papanicolaou smear	[d]	1	0	0
Enzymes	70–100	3	70	3
ESR	5	1–3	2	1.5
Amylase, lipase	2	1	0	0
Gall bladder x-ray	2	1	5	1
G.I. series	2	1	5	1
Urine culture	2	1	5	2
Blood sugar	0	0	100	2
Cholesterol	0	0	100	1.5
Triglycerides	0	0	100	1.5
Hemoglobin	0	0	15	12
Prothrombin time	0	0	15	30
Blood gases and pH	0	0	5	2

Note: The data presented in this table are based on the opinions of the fifteen primary-physician internists interviwed in the Yale study. These data refer to the period of the attack and a twelve-month period following the start of the attack.

a. Some of these tests and procedures are done during the period of hospitalization whereas others are done after the patient leaves the hospital but within the 12 month period following the start of the attack.

b. These data apply to the patients who survive an attack who should actually have had the test or procedure.

c. All patients, *conditions permitting*, should have a stool test for blood.

d. All females, *condition permitting*, should have a Papanicolaou smear.

note the marked similarity in values between the data in this table and those shown in Table 1. Perhaps this is because most internists consider themselves adequately trained in caring for patients with infarcts and therefore their care should be similar to that of the internist specializing in cardiology.

TABLE 3

Percentage of primary-physician internists' patients who survive an attack of myocardial infarction by kind of treatment required while under the care of primary-physician internists during the attack and within a twelve-month period following the start of the attack.

Treatment[a]	Percentage of patients requiring this kind of treatment
Bed rest	100
Diet therapy	100
I.V. fluids	100
Restricted activity	100
Stool softeners and/or cathartics	100
Narcotics	98
Sedation	90
Oxygen	75
Antiarrhythmic agents	50
Cardiotonic agents	33
Diuretics	33
Vasopressors	25
Anticoagulants	15
Antihypertensive therapy	5
Electrocardioversion	2
Physiotherapy	1
Pacemakers	
(a) temporary	5
(b) permanent	< 1

Note: The data presented in this table are based on the opinions of the fifteen primary-physician internists interviewed in the Yale study. These data refer to the period of the attack and a twelve-month period following the start of the attack.

a. Some treatments are performed in the hospital whereas others are done in the period following hospitalization.

Some of the visits indicated in the "treatment phase" section of Table 1 (and also of Table 4) are required either at home or at the attending physician's office *following* the period of hospitalization. The home visits—two visits for 80 per cent of the patients seen by primary-physician internists and slightly over four visits for 21 per cent of the cardiologists' patients—should be considered as part of

TABLE 4

Percentage of internist-cardiologists' patients who survive an attack of myocardial infarction who should be seen by internist-cardiologists for diagnosis, treatment, and follow-up, by location of visit, average number of visits per patient, and average time in minutes per visit per patient required during the attack and within a twelve-month period following the start of the attack.

Location of attendance[a]	Diagnostic phase[b]			Treatment phase[b]			Diagnostic and/or treatment phases combined[b]		
	Percentage of patients[e]	Average number of visits per patient[e]	Average time per visit per patient[e]	Percentage of patients[e]	Average number of visits per patient[e]	Average time per visit per patient[e]	Percentage of patients[e]	Average number of visits per patient[e]	Average time per visit per patient[e]
			(minutes)			(minutes)			(minutes)
All locations[d]	28	1.4	47	82	31.1	27	100	26.0	27
Internist-cardiologist's office	1	1.0	51	68	5.8	31	69	5.8	31
Patient's home	0	0	0	21	4.2	31	21	4.2	31
Hospital emergency room	2	1.0	45	0	0	0	2	1.0	45
Hospital in-patient	26	1.4	47	82	25.3	26	99	21.4	26

Note: The data presented in this table are based on the opinions of the six internist-cardiologists interviewed in the Yale study. These data refer to the period of the attack and a twelve-month period following the start of the attack.

a. A patient may be seen at more than one location for diagnosis and/or treatment

b. These data apply to patients who survive the attack who should have been seen at the particular location indicated for the phase of care specified.

c. The percentage of patients seen at a particular location for the phase of care specified is the percentage of all internist-cardiologist's patients who survive an attack of myocardial infarction. Not all the patients are seen during the diagnostic phase or during the treatment phase.

d. The all locations data are *not* the sums of the data shown for the specific locations as a patient can be seen at more than one location. Also, the all locations data are based on values for each of the specified locations that were carried to more decimal places than those shown in this table.

e. The average number of visits per patient and the average time per visit per patient refer to patients actually having visits with

124

the care necessary for the acute phase of the myocardial infarction. In like manner, a portion of the office visits—say one, two or possibly three visits out of the 4.5 mean number of visits with the primary-physician internist, or of the almost six visits with the cardiologist—should be allocated to the acute phase of the attack. The remainder of these office visits should be considered more or less as follow-up visits during the first twelve-month period of care.

The primary-physician internists who were interviewed stated that not many patients should require paramedical services. They indicated that approximately 4 per cent of myocardial infarction patients should require the services of visiting nurses, 1 per cent rehabilitation services, and less than 1 per cent social services. This may be considered by some persons as a low rate of utilization of paraprofessional services. One explanation for this may lie in the predominantly middle- and upper-class status of the physicians interviewed and in the kinds of patients that they are accustomed to having in their particular practices.

During each subsequent year that patients live following an attack of myocardial infarction, an average of 3.5 office visits (ranging from one to eight visits) per patient per year should be required with primary-physician internists. These visits should be of thirty minutes duration, on the average. These patients should have certain laboratory tests and procedures, including at least one urinalysis and one complete blood count during each year of follow-up. Those patients over forty years of age (and most myocardial infarction patients are over forty) should also have a chest film and an electrocardiogram. In addition, about 5 per cent of these myocardial infarction patients should have annual cholesterol and triglyceride determinations.

If patients should develop other myocardial infarcts, regardless of whether these occur during the first or subsequent years of treatment, the care required for the recurrent infarcts should be similar to that already described. As stated previously, all attacks of myocardial infarction require substantially the same diagnostic and therapeutic care with respect to professional–logistics, i.e., visits, time, consultations, tests, and procedures, and so forth.

As patients who survive an attack of myocardial infarction require an average of almost thirty-two visits of approximately twenty-three minutes average duration with primary-physician internists, slightly more than twelve hours of this type of physician's time is needed per surviving patient per acute phase of the attack. Moreover, each patient referred to an internist–cardiologist should require approximately the same amount of the cardiologist's time per attack as required with primary physicians, that is twelve hours.

For each full year of care, either between attacks or following the last attack, myocardial infarction patients should require, on the average, one and three-quarter hours of the primary-physician internists' time; this being based on an average of 3.5 visits each of about thirty minutes duration.

The previous descriptions of good care have not explicitly mentioned complications and coexisting diseases and conditions, although the professional–logistic data presented here do take into account complications that may be present. However, it may be that *other* diseases and conditions, if they exist, should or should not increase the total volume of services required, as a service may actually be provided simultaneously for more than one condition. Adjustments in the handling of the data can be made, if necessary, for these coexisting conditions.

Using this "per stage of the pathway" approach to the description of good care, it is possible to describe the "lifetime" care required for a group of patients that followed any one of the specific pathways shown in Figure 2. The care required for each specific pathway group becomes a function of how many attacks the group had, whether this is a group that survived the attack(s), the number of years between attacks (if the group concerns patients who have had more than one attack), and the average number of years that the group survived following the last attack. For the purposes of this paper, if the group is one that followed a pathway leading to one of the terminal states associated with the death of the patients *during the attack* of myocardial infarction, whether or not the death was due to the infarct (i.e., terminal states one, two, five, six, nine, or ten of Figure 2), an assumption has been made as follows: Patients who died *during* the course of active treatment of an attack of myocardial infarction required—during the period of the attack that they were alive—no fewer numbers of visits, tests, and procedures than required during the same time period by individuals who survived the attack. It is recognized that this assumption no doubt leads to an understatement of the total care needed for those people who died *during* the attack as they probably required more care during that same time period than did those patients who survived.

For the purpose of *illustration only* we will apply the previously described standards "per stage of the pathway" to data relating to myocardial infarction patients who have followed one or another of these pathways of disease, thus producing pathways of care for each of the various groups. To facilitate this presentation, data for certain terminal states will be combined. This will be done for terminal states one and two, five and six, and nine and ten, and for other terminal states involving third attacks. (Terminal states for third attacks are not shown in detail in Figure 2 but are included in Table 5.)

In spite of the difficulties inherent in trying to combine data obtained from several independent studies,[6] an attempt has been made here to do so in the hope of illustrating the methodology of preparing pathways of care. However, to simplify this task, data relating only to males fifty-five to sixty-four years of age at the time of their first myocardial infarct will be discussed. Sometimes, though, the necessary data applying specifically for this age–sex group were not available in the various publications used. Therefore, data for broader age groups and/or for both sexes were sometimes used as though the data applied directly to the fifty-five to sixty-four age group of males. Moreover, information about persons having three or more attacks was not actually presented in these published studies. In the absence of specific information, therefore, an assumption is being made for this paper that the rate of third attacks would be similar to that of second attacks, and so too would be the fatality

6. G. E. Dimond, "Prognosis of Men Returning to Work After First Myocardial Infarction," *Circulation* 23 (June, 1961): 881–85. S. Pell and D. A. D'Alonzo, "Immediate Mortality and Five-Year Survival of Employed Men With a First Myocardial Infarction," *The New England Journal of Medicine* 270 (April, 1964): 915–22. V. Van De Moortel and W. H. Kincaid, "Acute Coronary Occlusion: Time of Death," *PSA Reporter*, 7 (October, 1969), 1–2. E. Weinblatt, S. Shapiro, C. W. Frank, and R. V. Sager, "Prognosis of Men after First Myocardial Infarction: Mortality and First Recurrence in Relation to Selected Parameters," *American Journal of Public Health* 58 (August, 1968): 1329–54.

TABLE 5

Weighted average total number of visits and time required for the lifetime care of patients with primary-physician internists for the lifetime care of patients with myocardial infarction per male patient 55–64 years of age at onset of first attack of myocardial infarction.

Terminal state	Description of group	Percentage of all new MI cases	Weighted average total number of visits per patient in this group[a]	Weighted average total time per patient in this group[a] hour minutes
	1 attack only	74.0		
	Don't survive 1st attack	39.0		
1+2 (b)	die within 24 hours	32	1.4 } 3.94	0 46 } 1 hr. and
1+2 (b)	die between 1 day to 1 month	7	15.5 }	5 21 } 36 min.
	Survive 1st attack	35.0		
3 (b)	die between 1 month to 1 year	3	29.6	11 07
4 (b)	die between 2nd yr. to 15th yr. average of 9.5 years after start of first attack	32	61.4	26 59
	2 attack only group	21.5		
	Don't survive 2nd attack	13.0		
5+6 (b)	2 attacks in first year, die during 2nd attack	2	33.5	12 42
9+10(b)	2 attacks, 2nd attack occurs between 2nd and 15th year, dying during 2nd attack	11	65.3	28 35
	Survive 2nd attack	8.5		
7 (b)	2 attacks during 1st year, survive both attacks, die during first year	[d]	60.2	22 44
8 (b)	2 attacks within 1st year, survive both attacks, die between 2nd yr. to 15th yr. average of 9.5 years from start of 1st attack	1[d]	91.0	38 06
11(b)	2 attacks, 2nd attack occurs between 2nd to 15th yr., survive both attacks but die during year of 2nd attack, lived average of 9.5 yrs. after start of 1st attack	1	91.0	38 06

12(b)	2 attacks, 2nd attack occurs between 2nd to 15th year, die in some year subsequent to year of recovery from 2nd attack, lived average of 9.5 years after start of 1st attack	4.5			93.0	39	06
	3 attacks (or more)			6[d]			
	Don't survive 3rd attack						
(c)	3 attacks in 1st year, die during 3rd attack		2.2[d]		63.1	23	49
(c)	3 attacks, 2nd occurs between 1st to 15th year, 3rd between 2nd to 15th year, die during 3rd attack, lived average of 9.5 yrs. after start of 1st attack			2[d]	96.9	40	41
	Survive 3 attacks						
(c)	3 attacks 1st year, survive all 3 but die in 1st year		2.2[d]		79.8	33	50
(c)	3 attacks 1st year, survive all 3, die between 2nd to 15 yrs. live average of 9.5 years after start of 1st attack				120.6	49	13
(c)	3 attacks, 2nd occurs between 1st to 15th yr., 3rd between 2nd to 15th year, survive all three, live average of 9.5 years after start of 1st attack				124.1	50	58
	Weighted average for all MI cases	100.0%	100.0%	100.0%	42.6	18	18

Note: The data for the percentages of patients in each group were *estimated* from published sources. The percentages for third attacks were based on the assumption that third attacks would occur with the same frequency among survivors of second attacks as did second attacks among survivors of first attacks. A small percentage of patients will have more than three attacks over their lifetime. The data for the number of visits and time are based on the opinions of fifteen primary-physician internists interviewed in the Yale study.

a. These average totals are weighted totals based on the average number of years that a patient lived following the onset of the first MI.

b. Corresponds to terminal state shown on Figure 2.

c. These terminal states are not shown on Figure 2, but continuation points of pathways leading to these terminal states are shown by three asterisks on Figure 2.

d. Fewer than 1 per cent of the patients.

129

rate following these attacks. As none of the studies followed the men until all of them had died, it must be clearly understood that the two to fifteen year lifespan, and the average of 9.5 years used in this paper for those men who survive their first year of the disease, is only a rough estimate based on projecting the longevity of the study groups. By combining (or modifying) (a) data given in Table 1 for each attack of myocardial infarction, (b) the number of attacks sustained, (c) data for the interval of years between or following attacks, and (d) the average lifespan of a particular group, it was possible to calculate the weighted average total number of visits and time (in hours and minutes) required of primary-physician internists per patient for a particular pathway group. These averages are shown in Table 5. It is necessary to emphasize that these are only average values produced by using other average values. It should be recognized that for each pathway group, a range of values could have been estimated by using the range of data for each of the "per stage of the pathway" components. Although Table 5 refers only to primary-physician internists, similar estimates could be prepared for referral specialists such as cardiologists or vascular surgeons by using data specifically applicable to that kind of specialist.

For male patients ages fifty-five to sixty-four who died *during an attack*—whether the first, second, or third—an average value of almost four visits and slightly more than one and one-half hours of primary-physician internists' time per patient were used in various calculations for Table 5. These values are weighted averages resulting from the use of data applicable to the different proportions of patients dying within specified periods of time between the start of an attack of myocardial infarction and one month thereafter. Adjustments were also necessary for some of the calculations of Table 5 for the number of follow-up visits that a patient should have had when more than one attack was estimated to have occurred within a year, or when a person died during the year in which he survived an attack. In those cases, instead of using the almost thirty-two visits per patient for the particular year, slightly less than thirty visits were used in the calculations for that year per person per *attack*.

Table 5 shows the percentages of males, fifty-five to sixty-four years of age at the time of their first myocardial infarct, who theoretically have followed each of the pathways of disease leading to the various terminal states. Almost three-quarters of the men will have had only one attack, with over one-fifth having two attacks. The remaining men will have had three or more attacks—though this table only presents data in terms of three attacks. At this point it is necessary to indicate that these percentages are dependent upon which kinds of patients are included in the group being discussed. Specifically, the group of patients considered for this paper includes so-called "sudden death" patients as well as other myocardial infarction patients. If data were given in terms of myocardial infarcting patients *excluding* the sudden death group, the percentage of all starting patients that followed a specific pathway of disease would differ from that shown here. This would also be true if the starting group had been limited to hospitalized myocardial infarction patients only rather than to all myocardial infarction patients, whether hospitalized or not. The problem of silent (or unrecognized) infarcts must also be considered. The inclusion of this group would similarly alter the proportions of patients that follow one or another pathway.

For the population of myocardial infarction patients used here (including sudden deaths and nonhospitalized patients) about 44 per cent of the men having one or more attacks will have died within the first year. The largest proportion of these deaths (32 per cent) will have occurred during the first attack *and* within twenty-four hours.

With respect to all myocardial infarction patients the weighted average total number of visits and total time per patient varies according to the pathway of disease followed and ranges from less than two visits (three-quarters of an hour of the primary-physician's time) per patient who died within twenty-four hours of the first attack to approximately 124 visits, utilizing almost fifty-one hours of primary-physician internists' time per patient for those who survived three attacks and lived an average of 9.5 years from the time of the start of the first attack. Although Table 5 shows data only for visits and time a similar table could be produced for days of hospitalization, or any other item.

By using the proportions of patients following the various pathways and the data for visits and time for each specific pathway, it is possible to calculate the weighted average number of visits and time per patient having one or more attacks of myocardial infarction regardless of how long he survived. On the average, a male fifty-five years of age at the time of his first myocardial infarction should require during his remaining lifetime approximately forty-three visits for a total of more than eighteen hours of primary-physician time. If we accept an annual incidence rate for first myocardial infarctions of approximately 10 per 1,000 men of this age[7] and if we accept the present estimated number of civilian males, ages fifty-five to sixty-four, as 8,500,000,[8] then we can expect approximately 85,000 men to have their first myocardial infarction in a given year. These men collectively should require during their remaining lifetime 1,600,000 hours of primary-physician internists' time. This would be the equivalent of the full-time services of almost 725 internists, if we accept that internists, on the average, devote almost forty-six hours per week, forty-eight weeks per year to patient care.[9] Based on the assumption that the incidence, prevalence, mortality and repeat attack rates, and the length of survival do not change drastically from year to year, we could expect then to require this same number of physicians, 725, to care for the estimated yearly, almost 490,000 men with myocardial infarction—85,000 men having their first attack and being seen in their first year of care (first-year patients) and 400,000 or so men who have survived at least one year since the onset of their first attack, the carry-over group.[10]

Using various published estimates of incidence rates applicable to other age-sex specific groups (or a rate for all ages and both sexes combined) we could determine the number of new cases of myocardial infarction that would occur during a year for either

7. S. Shapiro, E. Weinblatt, C. W. Frank, and R. V. Sager, "Incidence of Coronary Heart Disease in a Population Insured for Medical Care (HIP)," *American Journal of Public Health* 59 (supplement to June, 1969): 1–101.

8. "Estimates of Civilian Resident Population of the United States by Age, Race, and Sex," United States Department of Commerce Bureau of Census, Series P-25, Number 416 (February, 1969), p. 16.

9. C. N. Theodore, G. E. Sutter, "A Report of the First Periodic Survey of Physicians," *Journal American Medical Association* 202 (November, 1967): 108–88.

10. This concept, and the formula used to derive the estimate of total cases and carry-over cases is discussed in reference cited in note 5.

those specific groups or for the population as a whole. Using data similar to that shown in Table 5, but applicable to each age–sex group (or for all ages combined), we could estimate the lifetime requirements in visits and time needed for those persons having a *first* myocardial infarction in a given year. Likewise, this information could be used to determine the amount of physicians' time required during any year for *all patients* (first-year and carry-over) having had at least one attack of myocardial infarction. Similar estimates could be made for visits and time required of other kinds of physicians, as well as estimates for facilities, e.g., hospital beds required. Finally, if costs per services (i.e., cost per visit or procedure performed by a particular kind of practitioner, cost of a hospital day or of a laboratory test, etc.) are applied to the number of each type of service that should be provided, or if the cost per required number of practitioners of each kind are used, an estimate can be made of the costs necessary for providing the care required by patients who have had one or more attacks of myocardial infarction. This estimate can be expressed either as the cost for providing care for a particular year, or as the cost for providing care over the "disease lifetime" of either an individual or of a group of persons needing that pathway of care.

Through the application of this method of expressing "lifetime" care required for groups of patients having a particular disease, it is hoped that a better understanding of patient care will result.

SUMMARY

A description of the total "good" care that people should receive for any specific disease or condition requires knowledge about the pathways of that disease and the standards of care applicable to the disease. The application of (a) the standards of good care to (b) the pathways of disease results in (c) descriptions of pathways of good care. The number of pathways for a given disease or condition varies with whether there can be repeated attacks (or flare-ups), whether the patients die during the attack, the number of such repeat attacks, and when these additional attacks occur.

A disease that can have only one attack has four major pathways:

two associated with patients who die during the attack, and two with those who survive the attack. A disease or condition having the potential of repeat attacks has the same four major pathways if there is only one attack. For the second attack, there are eight additional terminal states, four associated with death during the subsequent attack and the remaining four with patients who survive the second attack. The same logic can be applied to construct pathways for each additional attack beyond two.

Standards of good care for each of 170 adult diseases and 81 diseases affecting children are being prepared at Yale based on the opinions of active medical practitioners. Interviews are also being conducted with dentists and some pilot interviews were started with visiting nurses and social workers.

The interviews conducted with primary-physician internists and other types of medical specialists, such as cardiologists, gastroenterologists, and surgeons have resulted in the collection of data on location of visits, number of visits, tests, procedures, and consultations required for the description of good care for the prevention, diagnosis, treatment, and follow-up of patients for the particular disease or condition under discussion. Data are also being collected as to the percentage of patients to whom the previously described items refer. After editing and tabulating, these data are used in the formulation of indexes and standards of good care for each disease.

Tables have been presented in this paper showing the standards of good care for patients who survive attacks of myocardial infarction based on the opinions of fifteen primary-physician internists and six internist-cardiologists. Patients should have approximately the same degree of care for each attack—with regard to visits, time, and location of such care except for variations made necessary because of the specific requirements of individuals. Patients who survive an attack of myocardial infarction should receive on the average almost thirty-two visits per attack (each visit of more than twenty minutes duration, on the average) from primary-physician internists. Of these thirty-two visits, almost twenty-five should occur during the twenty-three days (mean value) of hospitalization. Additionally, patients should have approximately 3.5 visits, averaging about thirty minutes duration, for each year for which these patients survive an attack and do not have another attack. Thus the survived attacks should require on the average twelve hours of the primary-physician internist's time per patient during the first twelve months of care; and these patients should have on the average one and three quarter-hours of primary-physician internist's time per subsequent year following the attack provided that another attack does not occur. Some of the patients (from 10 per cent to almost 25 per cent) should be referred to cardiologists and should require about twenty-six visits averaging slightly less than one-half hour per attack, or about twelve hours of the cardiologist's time per surviving patient per attack.

The application of these "per stage of the pathway" standards to each of the pathways of disease leading to the various terminal states for myocardial infarction (similar to those shown in Figure 2) produce descriptions of good care for each pathway. Visits with primary-physician internists for the care necessitated by having had one or more attacks of myocardial infarction for men fifty-five to sixty-four years of age at the time of their first myocardial infarction ranges from about 1.5 visits to more than 124 visits. Seventy-four per cent of these men will have only one attack, about 22 per cent two attacks and the remainder three or more attacks. Those men (including sudden deaths) who die within twenty-four hours of their first attack will require on the average about three-quarters of an hour of the primary physician's time whereas those who survive *one* attack and live an average of 9.5 years from the start of the attack (32 per cent of all myocardial infarction patients) will require twenty-seven hours of the internist's time for the more than sixty-one visits required, on the average, over the patient's disease lifetime. Similar data are presented in this paper for each pathway of care.

Based on an estimated incidence rate of about 10 per 1,000 men fifty-five to sixty-four years of age, approximately 85,000 new cases of myocardial infarction will occur annually. These men will require a total of almost 1,600,000 hours of care while they are alive. This amounts to the full-time care of 725 internists. This is also equivalent to the yearly amount of care required by both new and old cases of myocardial infarction in men fifty-five to sixty-four years of age at the time of their first infarct. Annually, there will be approximately 85,000 new cases in this age–sex group. During any year there will be approximately 400,000 or so men who have survived at least one year since the onset of the first attack.

Thus, through the application of (a) data on professional–logistics, such as number of visits, time per visit, tests, and procedures required to (b) data on incidence and prevalence of disease, it is possible to (c) estimate the manpower required to provide care for patients with a particular disease. When these estimates are combined (either disease by disease, or by groups of diseases) estimates can be arrived at for total manpower needs. With appropriate application of data on costs per service or costs per type of provider, estimates can be made of the expenditures that would be required in order to provide good care for all people.

The studies on Standards of Medical Care described in this paper are under the general direction of Dr. I. S. Falk. Dr. Paul H. Lavietes and Dr. Philip K. Bondy are clinical co-chairmen of the medical studies.

The author wishes to express his thanks to the other staff members, Mrs. Jean Heston, Research Associate in Public Health (Medical Care) and Mrs. Mary Gardner, Associate in Research (Medical Care), for their assistance in this study and to the following physicians whose opinions have been used at various times throughout the study though not necessarily for the disease discussed in this paper.

PARTICIPATING PHYSICIANS
YALE FACULTY OF MEDICINE*

Adult Medicine

Adams, Elisabeth C.
Bender, Morton
Bishop, Courtney C.
Bondy, Philip K.
Brodoff, Murray
Burrow, Gerald N.
Carpinella, Michael J.
Chernoff, Hyman M.

Chetrick, Allen
Cipriano, Anthony P.
Cole, Jack W.
Coleman, Jules V.
Corradino, Charles L.
Dwyer, Hugh L., Jr.
Evans, Theodore S.
Fazzone, Philip R.

*Member of the Yale Faculty of Medicine at the time of the interviews.

Fleck, Stephen
Gallaher, William H.
Gordon, Martin E.
Gordon, Robert S.
Harris, Benedict R.
Hogan, Gilbert F.
Houlihan, Robert K.
Johnson, Kenneth G.
Jordan, Robert H.
Kaetz, Harvey W.
Kushlan, Samuel D.
Landau, S. Jack
Lavietes, Paul H.
Lavietes, Stanley R.
Levy, Lewis L.
Lewis, Herbert D.
Lillian, Marvin
Mignone, Joseph

Milles, Saul S.
Moench, John C.
Molumphy, Paul E.
Morgan, Walter S.
Nahum, Louis H.
Piccolo, Pasquale A.
Quilligan, Edward J.
Rilance, Arnold B.
Roth, Oscar S.
Scherr, Edward H.
Scherr, Edward S.
Selzer, Richard A.
Spinner, Samuel
Swift, William E.
Van Eck, William F.
White, Robert M.
Zimmerman, Martin P.

Pediatric Medicine

Baratz, Merrill A.
Beloff, Jerome S.
Clement, David H.
Cook, Charles D.
Culotta, Charles S.
Cunningham, Peter R.
Goldstein, Paul S.
Granger, Richard H.
Gruskay, Frank L.
Hurwitz, Sidney
Krassner, Leonard S.
Krosnick, Morris Y.

Landwirth, Julius
Lattanzi, William E.
McAlenney, Paul F.
Mermann, Alan C.
Morrison, John B.
Pearson, R. J. C.
Shelling, Richard L.
Stein, Michael L.
Stilson, Carter
Wakeman, Edward T.
Wessel, Morris A.
Wilson, William R.

This investigation is supported in part by a grant (CRD #332) from the Social and Rehabilitation Service and the Social Security Administration, United States Department of Health, Education and Welfare, Washington, D.C. The earlier phases of the study were supported in part by a grant (CH00037) from the Division of Community Health Service, Public Health Service.

137

Need for More Effective Use of Health Personnel

by DARREL J. MASE

PRESIDENT JOHNSON in his message to Congress relative to the aged on January 23, 1967, pointed out that there were at that time 19 million Americans sixty-five years of age or over, a number equal to the combined populations of twenty of the states. One out of every ten citizens was in this age group, or more than twice as many as a half century ago. He then went on to point out that with the increasing growth in scientific knowledge the life span can be expected to stretch even farther. President Johnson further emphasized that too often the wisdom and experience of our senior citizens is lost or ignored. Many who are able and willing to work suffer the bitter rebutt of arbitrary and unjust job discrimination. The President mentioned that in 1965 the Congress had enacted into law two measures for older Americans—Medicare and the Older Americans Act—which undertake to provide for the medical care of a portion of our population. These and other national developments stress the need of changing the delivery of health care and of better utilization of health manpower.

Arnold Toynbee said fifteen years ago something to the effect that the twentieth century will be chiefly remembered as an age in which the human society dared to think of the welfare of the whole human race. That day has arrived, as society demands that good

138

health care and well-being for all and comprehensive rehabilitation services for those with illnesses and disabilities be among the rights and privileges of all citizens. This decision, without adequate time to prepare the needed manpower, to alter the delivery of health care systems, and to provide the needed facilities for this extension of health care, provides a challenge that demands thoughtful and considered judgments.

Senior citizens can help to bring about this necessary change which cannot and will not be brought about by organized medicine or by hospital administrators. It can and will only be brought about by citizens. There is a knowledgeable group, a very intelligent group, of senior citizens that can be given a better life, and they can give society a better life if their energies can be drawn to some changes that are inevitable. This task is most important to you and therefore to the senior citizens you represent because even though they have Medicare they do not have health care; they will not have health care until it can be delivered without the danger of our health care system breaking down.

The continuing extension of years of life is quite assured. A new problem of human experience has appeared in our western world. No culture in previous history has ever had such a high proportion of its people past middle age. The problem is primarily related to four factors, economic, social, medical, and personal. All of us want to live a long time but we don't want to get older. Yet aging is quite inseparable from life. The process of aging takes place from the day we're born. What we need to consider along with extending life is how to make it a full and happy experience throughout whatever years God chooses to give us. What can be done not only to keep people alive but to give them a chance to live and to be productive members of society?

We need to ask ourselves the question, "How old is old?" Perhaps we need to rewrite the question to read "Old, with respect to what performance?" Retirement is expected in relation to the years persons have lived rather than in relation to their needs or capacities. Some people are quite old at thirty and others are quite young at seventy-five. It is interesting that the destiny of our society may be guided by congressmen, legislators, and supreme court justices whose age is no matter, but school teachers, social workers, and people in other occupations seem to wear out quickly. Age is not measurable by years but by attributes. It is estimated that 64 per cent of the world's great achievements have been accomplished by men who have passed their sixtieth year. Johann von Goethe started his dramatic poem at age twenty and finished it at eighty-three. Even if the circumstances of employment make it impossible for a man or woman to continue after the pensionable age is completed, this must not be the end of the road.

There are opportunities to serve in the field of health, where manpower is needed and where the knowledge, skills, and experiences of senior citizens can contribute much. Basically (and unfortunately) a large portion of society is organized to satisfy the wants of the young and makes relatively little provision even yet for meeting the needs of the aged. Too often the aged are tolerated and too seldom valued. It is my belief that young people should be taught early how to grow old. Senior citizens could do much of this teaching. They could share their experiences and help people to grow old. We know, but do we apply the knowledge? Merely the realm of the physical provides examples. Repeated insults to the human machine in earlier life such as infections, injuries, strains, chronic malnutrition, alcoholism, smoking, drug addiction, obesity, shock, and emotional turbulence cause changes in the body cells which are conducive to aging.

Just what are the distinguishing attributes of various age groups? Youth is marked by resiliency, strength, and mobility. Maturity shows balance, precision, and achievement. The good qualities of old age are thoroughness, steadiness, dependability, wisdom. One thing remains irrevocably fixed, and this is that our allotment of time at age sixty-five is just what it was at fifteen—twenty-four hours a day. It behooves us to use every hour of that in accord with the wisdom we have picked up along the way. We can make this world a better place to live in as well as satisfy the needs of senior citizens.

Now to my challenge to you. I urge that you help the senior citizens that you represent in the necessary understanding, cooperation, personal effort to bring about more effective utilization of health personnel and improved systems of delivery of health care. *Fortune* Magazine of January, 1970, reaffirms the mess we're in, and it is a mess. Five articles are included in a special section entitled, "Our Ailing Medical System." It begins by stating: "American medicine, the pride of the nation for many years, stands now on the brink of chaos. . . . much of U.S. medical care, particularly the everyday business of preventing and treating routine illnesses, is inferior in quality, wastefully dispensed, and inequitably financed.

"Whether poor or not, most Americans are badly served by the obsolete, overstrained medical system that has grown up around them helter-skelter. . . . In the words of the two federal officials who are the most concerned—Secretary Robert H. Finch of Health, Education, and Welfare, and his Assistant Secretary of Health, Dr. Roger O. Egeberg—'This nation is faced with a breakdown in the delivery of health care unless immediate concerted action is taken by government and the private sector.'"

This issue of *Fortune* Magazine is suggested reading for all senior citizens as part of their continuing education. It helps to see what we are up against. The articles do not provide the answers we need but they help us to understand the problem; the problem must be understood before solutions can be sought. Health is our second largest industry, with total public and private expenditures under public programs in 1968–69 of a little over 60 billion dollars. In 1900 in the United States there was one supportive person in a health occupation or profession for each physician. Today the ratio is thirteen to one. By 1975 it is anticipated that the ratio will necessarily be twenty-five to one. Dr. Lowell T. Coggeshall stated in his report to the Executive Council of the Association of American Medical Colleges in 1965 that "increasing physician productivity is probably the most important step required to alleviate the growing physician 'shortage.' This will require delegating tasks to others."

The technological developments that are moving into our laboratories and the number of people that are, for instance, in the operating room for open heart surgery or for body transplants have caused this great increase. There is a whole new array of kinds of health personnel that have to be prepared for the marketplace. Our eleven-year old College of Health Related Professions may be taken as an illustration. The University of Florida was the first university to have a college of health related professions and a medical

141

college jointly integrated in the larger administrative structure of a health center. Since the new conception—a college of health related professions within the University—was an experiment, it was tolerated but not well supported. However, in 1965, John Gardner, then Secretary of Health, Education and Welfare, in testimony before a congressional committee, indicated that one of the things needed to meet the health manpower mandate was colleges such as the College of Health Relation Professions at the University of Florida. Suddenly it became a model for the nation. However, by April, 1967, there were still only twelve similar administrative structures in the country, each with three or more degree programs.

Currently the College of Health Related Professions is composed of eight departments: (1) Department of Medical Technology, leading to the Bachelor of Science in Medical Technology; (2) Department of Occupational Therapy, leading to the degree Bachelor of Science in Occupational Therapy; (3) Department of Physical Therapy, leading to the degree Bachelor of Science in Physical Therapy; (4) Department of Rehabilitation Counseling, leading to the degree Master of Rehabilitation Counseling; (5) Department of Clinical Psychology which is responsible for the teaching of specialized courses in clinical psychology, and for providing intern and practicum experiences in clinical psychology for the Department of Psychology, College of Arts and Sciences; (6) Department of Communicative Disorders which is responsible for complementing and supplementing the Department of Speech, College of Arts and Sciences, in the training of speech pathologists and audiologists and for offering training to post-doctoral students who wish to work in medical settings; (7) Department of Health and Hospital Administration in which students work for the Master's Degree in Business Administration with a specialization in health and hospital administration; and (8) Rehabilitation Research Institute. This institute is supported by a grant from the Rehabilitation Services Administration, of the Social and Rehabilitation Services, United States Department of Health, Education, and Welfare. Its responsibility is to conduct core research in rehabilitation, to assist and cooperate with various departments within the college and health center in designing and carrying out research, and to promote the rehabilitation research movement in the southeastern region.

142

Other programs which were approved by the former Board of Control when space could be made available were for bachelor's degrees for medical record librarians, and radiological technologists, and a master's degree in medical illustration. Still other programs which must be established are for social workers at the bachelor's and master's level, and dental hygienists at the bachelor's degree level. Teacher training programs in dental hygiene and dental assisting are also anticipated. Other health occupations which have received attention by this college include: medical dietitians, public health nutritionists, psychological assistants, speech pathology assistants, audiology assistants, mental health workers, physician assistants, orthoptists, and prosthetists. These and many other health personnel will be needed if we meet society's commitment to health. Those to be prepared for these and other health careers should receive their education and training in settings where physicians and dentists are being prepared.

The major goals of the College of Health Related Professions at the University of Florida include the following: (1) To prepare health personnel as need is indicated with bachelor's and graduate degrees. (2) To prepare staff to teach in junior colleges and to assist these colleges in preparing those for the health careers at that level. (3) To administer a program of health related services to patients in the teaching hospital and clinics, and to relate to the veterans administration hospital and to other community health facilities in this section of the state as a basis for providing the clinical experiences necessary by those the college represents but as well those represented by the J. Hillis Miller Health Center and the University of Florida. (4) To develop programs of continuing education for those practicing the health occupations represented by the college. (5) To encourage and administer a program of research in specific areas of health and rehabilitation.

The long range plans indicate that the academic faculty should move from the thirty-eight now on the staff at the present time to 101 in 1977–78. The total staff would increase from 84 at the present time to 202 in 1977–78. Students would increase from 396 in the fall of 1967 to 959 in 1977–78. This does not include staff for the dental hygiene and the dental assistant programs as they are included at this time in the projections of the College of Dentistry.

People are kept in college longer now than in times past. There are 1,150 junior colleges in the United States. In recent years an average of one new junior college is being built every ten days. We have now extended general education to fourteen grades by the advent of the junior college concept. It seems that, to keep a reasonable proportion of the population reasonably occupied, people must be retained in college longer, must be retired earlier, and the nation must be at war or preparing for war. By 1975, 80 per cent of all high school graduates may go on to college. The interweaving of the commitment to advanced education for a large segment of youth, the demand for extended health care services, and the potential of the socioeconomic base stimulate all responsible agencies and groups to respond creatively. Planning without action is futile and action without planning is fatal. Furthermore, action must benefit the people that are here right now, not their putative grandchildren.

In order to share ideas and analyze the situation, representatives of the thirteen colleges and universities with established programs met at Ohio State University in April of 1967. At that meeting it was decided that an association was needed to speak as a united voice in behalf of the many and varied health occupations and professions. Four months later, the Association of Schools of Allied Health Professions was officially formed. A few weeks later, the staff of the Kellogg Foundation responded to the Association's need for a central office in Washington, D.C. The Association could then begin to speak with one united interdisciplinary voice in behalf of patients and patient needs. In September, 1968, the first annual meeting elicited 433 registrants from 43 states, over a third of whom were physicians. The association is totally interdisciplinary and speaks in behalf of those patients and those individuals who need attention and health care. This past year, the association has struggled to find ways and means to give voting privileges to junior colleges, to 125 different organizations and associations that are interested in health, and to some one thousand individual members who had joined the association.

Senior citizens should be solicited to support a cause in respect to better delivery of health care and better utilization of health manpower. When the cause is on the behalf of people and not on behalf of personal aggrandizement and personal interests, your voice can be heard. To get things done in this societal pattern where scientific knowledge doubles every eighteen months, forces must be to bring about the necessary changes or else many people will suffer. But to this day, we seem to feel that adequate health care and adequate delivery of health care will somehow be provided with little attention from us.

One or two things should be interpreted to your senior citizens—things that are happening that ought to be stopped or that ought to be directed properly. Hospitals have classically trained a great many supportive people to medicine on certificate and diploma programs. The large majority of the nurses have come from diploma schools which consume three years. A diploma school nurse from a hospital gains no academic credit, no way to fit into the mainstream of education today, and no upward mobility to other things. Hospitals must phase out such training, and the training must be fitted into academic units—vocational schools, technical schools, junior colleges, and universities. The hospitals and other health facilities should provide the clinical training experiences, but the education and training is a job for academia unless we want to prepare a still greater group of disadvantaged, underprivileged people in the health field. Graduates must be able members of society. Hospitals have been classically able to provide training to groups of people at the lower wage level that win dead-end jobs. But dead-end jobs do not spell democracy now and neither will they in societies in the future. People with motivation, desire, ability, must have an opportunity to go on to other and better opportunities. We have not built this mobility into our training system.

Medicare, medicaid, and other third party payers are increasing the pressure to urge that hospitals not be permitted to write off education and training costs to patient fees. More and more, funding through state and federal agencies and private foundations for those in the health occupations and professions will be through academic units. This change solves many problems, not the least of which is the issue of career mobility. Three years in a hospital nurses' training program with no academic credits to transfer for any kind of a degree—associate, bachelor's, or anything else—does not enhance mobility or respectability in our mobile society. On the

Health Care Services for the Aged

other hand, two years in a junior college with a mixture of one year of general education and a year of specialization which qualifies a student to pass the registered nurse examination, does fit the pattern of mobility as the student would also have an associate's degree in addition to her R.N. degree.

The same criticism can be applied to nearly all of the hospital-based programs of preparation of personnel. The real question is can the colleges, junior colleges, and universities do as well in preparing allied health personnel as the hospitals have done and with enhanced respectability and mobility? It is possible, with the cooperation and support of the hospitals and other health facilities—if these facilities will provide opportunities for the necessary clinical training experiences. Those in the hospitals must understand that the job they have done is not the same as that which must be done by our various academic programs. Specifically, hospitals have never been interested in supplying the larger marketplace with personnel in the various health areas, but rather they have trained their own personnel in order to meet their own needs. They were satisfied to have small classes which were just large enough to meet their basic needs. Academic units, on the other hand, cannot run classes that provide only one, two, or three graduates a year. But they can run larger programs that accommodate for mobility and that accommodate the demand for needed health personnel. This unique capacity necessitates planning and action which has not been accomplished in the past. It may mean that each community which has a hospital which has trained its health personnel cannot simply transfer to academic programs in their educational, vocational, or junior college for the same health personnel. It means that states and regions must decide what is the best utilization of the education and training resources to obtain the needed health manpower. This will necessitate a change in the philosophy and thinking of those in the hospitals and in the communities in the ways their efforts are spent generating health manpower to provide the needed services.

Senior citizens have the time to help in the planning for who does what in the technical vocational schools, junior colleges, colleges, and universities so that duplication of programs and gaps in programs will both be avoided.

146

Effective use of manpower demands not only that physicians
learn to delegate tasks to others but also clinical psychologists,
speech pathologists, physical therapists, occupational therapists,
and a host of others. This reassignment of duties seems easy but is
inhibited by complacency in the status quo. In the first chapter in
his book, *No Easy Victories,* John W. Gardner states that, "Even excellent institutions run by excellent human beings are inherently
sluggish, *not* hungry for innovation, *not* quick to respond to human
needs, *not* eager to reshape themselves to meet the challenges of
the times. I am not suggesting a polarity between men and their
institutions—men eager for change, their institutions blocking it. The
institutions are run by men. And often those who appear most eager
for change oppose it most stubbornly when their own institutions are
involved. I give you the university professor, a great friend of
change provided it doesn't affect the patterns of academic life. His
motto is, 'Innovate away from home.' We are going to have to do a
far more imaginative and aggressive job renewing, redesigning, and
revitalizing our institutions, if we are to meet the requirements of
today."

Somehow expressions of the better utilization of manpower seem
to be interpreted to mean more of the same. Projections in respect
to the needs for more physicians, more clinical psychologists, more
of all health personnel is almost universally on the basis that those
in the health occupations and professions will do what they have
been doing, whatever their health specialty. We went to school to
learn the knowledge and skills necessary to begin practicing our
specialty. We also were taught that what we had was ours and ours
alone to use. We were not taught that some of these knowledges
and skills could be, and should be, delegated to others, to be applied
under our supervision.

The health ladder, to provide mobility which we hear so much
about, has not been as effective. In health care, the enterprise is
dominated by a relatively small group of professionals at the top
of the pyramid—physicians, administrators, clinical psychologists,
and others with nine plus years beyond high school. Then a thin
line is found down to bachelor's degree people with three years,
and this largely represents the three-year hospital based program
for training. The lower base of the pyramid includes the aides and

147

attendants with no formalized preparation. The need is apparent for middle manpower in the largely uninhabited intermediate areas where mobility is currently low and often not possible. An orderly seldom becomes a nurse; a nurse almost never a doctor. Because of low mobility and generally low pay in the bottom layers, lower layers have often been filled with individuals with limited intellectual capacity and small educational achievements. Those from the minority groups have had their access to more promising jobs hampered or blocked, but if there is one thing clear today, it is that minorities are not going to continue to be shunted into low-level dead-end jobs. I urge you to help senior citizens to accept and support the changes in the distribution of health care manpower and services. I urge you to help senior citizens to become very actively engaged in this changing delivery system of health care, for instance, the "hospital" that Anne Somers talked about earlier in this book. To accomplish the reality of this new concept, it would be better to come up with another term because hospital does not connote the totality of services and functions that must be performed.

The existentialism of professional groups makes it difficult to bring about these changes in any other way. Some professional people and administrators speak and write about preparing "sub-professional" people in the community junior colleges. The term subprofessional does not imply dignity, belongingness, neededness. When used by professionals, it somehow implies "everyone below me," and to the person whom we wish to prepare for the important role of assisting with the health care and treatment of our citizenry, it somehow implies "in the gutter if not in the sewer and no way to get out."

Another term which does not seem to give a desirable connotation in describing those in the health occupations is "paramedical." *Dorland's American Illustrated Medical Dictionary* defines "para" as a prefix meaning *"beside, beyond, accessory to, apart from, against."* Webster's offers, "by the side of, beside, along side of, by, *past, beyond, to one side, aside from, amiss."* Six of these terms connote the concept desired, while eight give a different meaning. Better terms than "sub-professional" and "paramedical" would be "allied," "associated," or "health related," professions. Let us use words and descriptive phrases which help us achieve our goals rather than militate against them.

At the American Public Health Association meeting in San Francisco in November, I presented a paper on "Mindpower Utilization." Mindpower utilization implies that the individual with advanced education and training will always supervise and direct the activities of the individual with less preparation. Such a delegation of responsibilities would lead to efficient utilization of mindpower, would maintain quality services, and would make for a better balance of the lopsided distribution of those in the health occupations. There *can* and *must* be dignity at each level of preparation and in each job to be performed.

The creed of Alcoholics Anonymous, drawn from the words of Reinhold Niebuhr, are suitable to use in closing: "God, grant me the serenity to accept the things I cannot change; the courage to change the things that I can, and the wisdom to know the difference." And I pray that you will help the senior citizens you represent to become actively involved with a system of delivery of health care and better utilization of manpower; otherwise, Medicare or no Medicare, they will not receive health care.